THE ULTIMATE GUIDE TO FATTY LIVER

2000 DAYS OF EASY AND ECONOMICAL MEALS TO DETOXIFY YOUR LIVER WITHOUT STRESS. REVERSE FATTY LIVER WITHOUT TOO MANY SACRIFICES WITH QUICK AND TASTY RECIPES, TO START AGAIN WITH ENERGY AND VITALITY. INCLUDES 30-DAY MEAL PLAN.

CHRIS MARSHALL

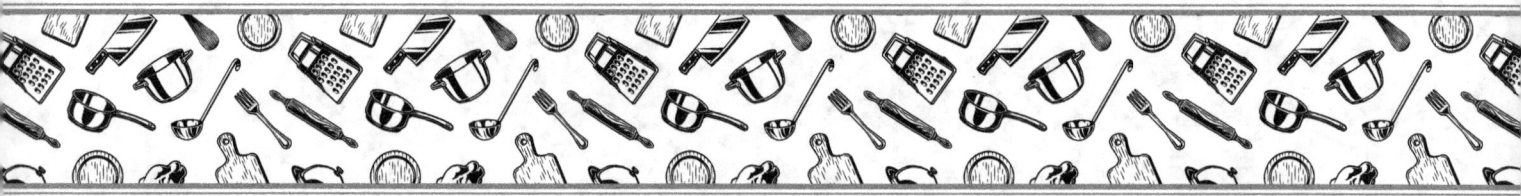

© **Copyright 2024: CHRIS MARSHALL All rights reserved.**

The content contained within this book may not be reproduced, duplicated, or transmitted without direct written permission from the author or the publisher.

Under no circumstances will any blame or legal responsibility be held against the publisher, or author, for any damages, reparation, or monetary loss due to the information contained within this book. Either directly or indirectly.

Legal Notice:

This book is copyright protected. This book is only for personal use. You cannot amend, distribute, sell, use, quote, or paraphrase any part, or the content within this book, without the author's or publisher's consent.

Disclaimer Notice:

Please note the information contained within this document is for educational and entertainment purposes only. All effort has been executed to present accurate, up-to-date, and reliable, complete information. No warranties of any kind are declared or implied. Readers acknowledge that the author does not render legal, financial, medical, or professional advice. The content within this book has been derived from various sources. Please consult a licensed professional before attempting any techniques outlined in this book.

By reading this document, the reader agrees that under no circumstances is the author responsible for any direct or indirect losses incurred due to the use of the information contained within this document, including, but not limited to, errors, omissions, or inaccuracies.

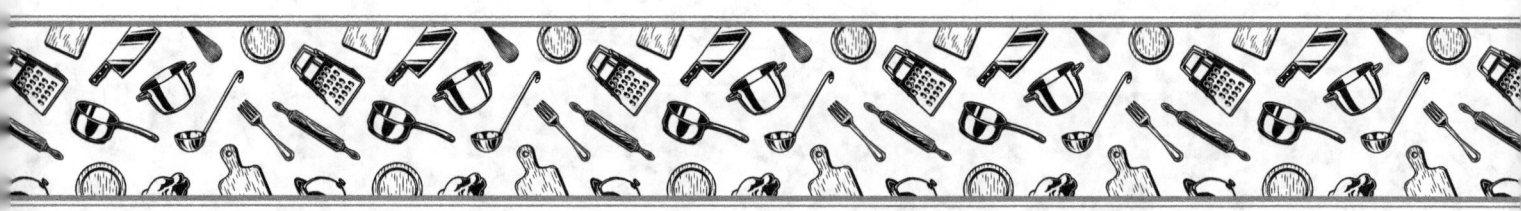

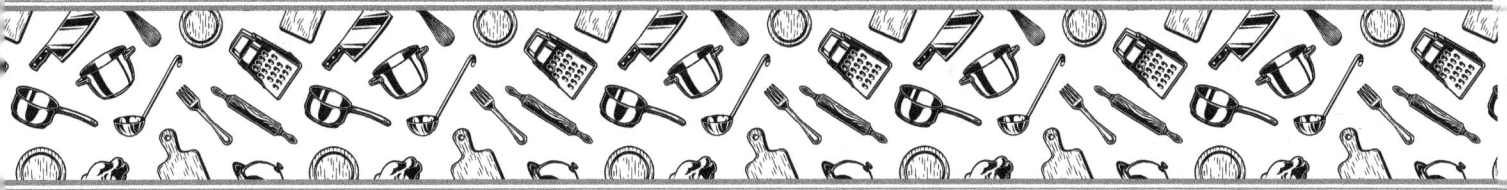

TABLE OF CONTENT

AUTHOR INFORMATION 7
INTRODUCTION 10
   Calculate Your Fatty Liver Index 10

BREAKFAST

SWEET BREAKFASTS 13
   1. Oat and Fruit Smoothie (Vegan) 13
   2. Greek Yogurt with Honey and Almonds (Vegetarian) 13
   3. Quinoa Porridge with Fruit (Vegan) 14
   4. Banana and Coconut Muffins (Vegetarian) 14
   5. Cinnamon and Apple Muffins (Vegetarian) 16

SAVORY BREAKFASTS 17
   6. Scrambled Eggs with Spinach and Tomatoes (Vegetarian) 17
   7. Avocado and Egg Toast (Vegetarian) 18
   8. Spinach and Tomato Omelette (Vegetarian) 19
   9. Sweet Potato Pancakes (Vegetarian) 20
   10. Buckwheat Pancakes with Yogurt and Fresh Fruit (Vegetarian) 21
   11. Chickpea Cream and Tomato Toast (Vegetarian) 22

MEAT-BASED DISHES 23
   12. Chicken Curry with Brown Rice 23
   13. Turkey Meatloaf with Mashed Potatoes and Carrots 24
   14. Chicken alla Pizzaiola with Brown Rice 25
   15. Quinoa Salad with Grilled Chicken 26
   16. Couscous with Chicken Curry 27
   17. Whole Wheat Tagliatelle with Turkey and Mushroom Sauce 28
   18. Lemon Chicken with Grilled Asparagus 29
   19. Turkey Taco Bowl with Brown Rice 30
   20. Beef Stew with Vegetables: 31
   21. Lean Beef Chili 32
   22. Turkey and Black Bean Chili 33
   23. Baked Chicken Meatballs with Sweet Potatoes 34
   24. Veal Steak with Arugula and Tomato Salad 35

FISH-BASED DISHES 36
   25. Grilled Salmon with Lemon and Caper Sauce 36
   26. Steamed Salmon with Zucchini Risotto 37
   27. Tuna and Orzo Salad 37
   28. Tuna and Tomato Pasta Salad 38
   29. Salmon Meatballs with Brown Rice and Grilled Vegetables 39

30. Lemon Shrimp Risotto 40
31. Couscous Salad with Smoked Salmon 41
32. Shrimp and Pineapple Skewers with Brown Rice 42
33. Salmon with Almond Crust and Steamed Broccoli 43
34. Grilled Swordfish with Black Bean Salad 43
35. Octopus Salad with Tomatoes and Olives 44

VEGAN AND VEGETARIAN DISHES 45

36. Barley and Chickpea Salad 45
37. Tofu Curry with Brown Rice 46
38. Roasted Vegetable Couscous 46
39. Zucchini Noodles with Avocado Pesto 47
40. Lentil Taco 47
41. Grilled Vegetable Wrap 48
42. Corn Tortillas with Beans and Salsa 48

SOUPS AND BROTHS 49

43. Vegetable Soup 49
44. Lentil Soup 50
45. Minestrone with Barley 50
46. Pumpkin and Carrot Soup 51
47. Pea and Mint Soup 51
48. Spinach and Potato Soup 52
49. Caramelized Onion Soup 52
50. Lentil and Tomato Soup 53
51. Pumpkin and Ginger Soup 54
52. Cauliflower and Curry Soup 55

SALADS AND SIDES

SALADS 57

53. Spinach and Strawberry Salad 57
54. Quinoa Salad with Roasted Vegetables 57
55. Black Bean and Corn Salad 57
56. Chickpea and Tomato Salad 58
57. Cucumber and Melon Salad 58
58. Beet and Cucumber Salad 58
59. Farro Salad with Cherry Tomatoes and Olives 59
60. Roasted Tomato and Cucumber Salad 59
61. Couscous and Vegetable Salad 59
62. Green Bean and Almond Salad 59

SIDE DISHES 60

63. Chickpea and Tomato Salad 60
64. Sautéed Spinach with Garlic and Lemon 60
65. Roasted Sweet Potatoes 60
66. Steamed Broccoli with Almonds 61
67. Quinoa and Vegetable Salad 61
68. Cauliflower Gratin 61
69. Beet and Chickpea Salad 61
70. Cucumber and Avocado Salad 62
71. Grilled Zucchini with Basil Pesto 62
72. Green Beans with Almonds and Lemon 62
73. Arugula and Strawberry Salad 63
74. Grilled Eggplant with Parsley Pesto 63
75. Artichokes Gratin with Breadcrumbs and Lemon 63

FAST FUEL FAST FOOD 64

76. Grilled Chicken Sandwich and Baked Potato Chips 64
77. Vegetarian Sandwich with Hummus and Baked Potato Chips 65
78. Turkey Burger Sandwich with Roasted Potato Wedges 66
79. BLT Sandwich with Paprika Potato Chips 67
80. Philly Cheese Steak Sandwich with Thyme Potato Wedges 68

PIZZAS

DOUGH 70
- 81. Whole Wheat Pizza Dough 70
- 82. Chickpea Flour Pizza Dough 70
- 83. Oat Flour Pizza Dough 71
- 84. Corn Flour Pizza Dough 71
- 85. Coconut Flour Pizza Dough 71
- 86. Buckwheat Flour Pizza Dough 72
- 87. Light Margherita Pizza 72
- 88. Vegetarian Pizza with Grilled Vegetables 73
- 89. Pizza with Chicken and Spinach 73
- 90. Pizza with Tuna and Capers 74
- 91. Pizza with Mushrooms and Arugula 74
- 92. Pizza with Smoked Salmon and Avocado 75
- 93. Pizza with Tomatoes and Fresh Basil 75
- 94. Pizza with Mixed Mushrooms and Caramelized Onions 76
- 95. Pizza with Shrimp and Arugula Pesto 76
- 96. Pizza with Mushrooms and Spinach 77

CUISINES FROM AROUND THE WORLD

ITALIAN RECIPES 79
- 97. Spaghetti alla Puttanesca 79

CHICKEN CACCIATORE 80
- 98. Chicken Cacciatore 80
- 99. Eggplant Parmigiana Light 81
- 100. Whole Wheat Pasta with Tomato and Basil 82
- 101. Caprese Salad 83
- 102. Bruschetta with Cherry Tomatoes and Basil 83
- 103. Whole Wheat Linguine with Avocado Sauce 84

FRENCH RECIPES 85
- 104. Ratatouille 85
- 105. Coq au Vin (Chicken in Wine) 86
- 106. Bouillabaisse (Fish Soup) 87
- 107. Cassoulet 87
- 108. Quiche with Vegetables 88
- 109. Beef Bourguignon 89

GREEK RECIPES 90
- 110. Chicken Souvlaki with Tzatziki 90
- 111. Greek Salad 91
- 112. Melitzanosalata 91
- 113. Spanakopita 92
- 114. Fasolada (Bean Soup) 93
- 115. Chickpea Tzatziki 93

CHINESE RECIPES 94
- 116. Vegetable Fried Rice 94
- 117. Chicken and Corn Soup: 95
- 118. Cabbage and Carrot Salad: 95
- 119. Steamed Orange Chicken 96
- 120. Stir-Fried Tofu with Vegetables 96
- 121. Steamed Chinese Dumplings with Spinach and Mushroom Filling 97
- 122. Sautéed Zucchini Noodles with Chicken and Soy Sauce 98
- 123. Peking Duck with Vegetables 99

JAPANESE RECIPES 100
- 124. Preparation of Sushi Rice 100
- 125. Vegetarian Sushi Rolls: 101

- 126. Sauteed Edamame 101
- 127. Yakitori Chicken with Reduced Teriyaki Sauce 102
- 128. Steamed Vegetarian Gyoza 102
- 129. Miso Soup with Tofu and Seaweed 103
- 130. Japanese Ramen 103
- 131. Miso Soup with Tofu and Seaweed (for one person) 103

SNACK 104
- 132. Fruit Salad 104
- 133. Greek Yogurt with Blueberries and Almonds 104
- 134. Homemade Cereal Bars 105
- 135. Whole Grain Crackers with Avocado 105
- 136. Apple and Cinnamon Muffins 106
- 137. Chocolate Avocado Mousse 106
- 138. Fruit and Nut Bars 107
- 139. Peanut Butter and Rice Crispy Bars 107

DESSERT 108
- 140. Banana and Cocoa Ice Cream 108
- 141. Baked Pears with Cinnamon and Walnuts 108
- 142. Coconut and Mixed Berry Chia Pudding 109
- 143. Sugar-Free Apple Cake 109
- 144. Lemon Sorbet 110
- 145. Coconut and Berry Panna Cotta 110
- 146. Protein Banana Ice Cream 111
- 147. Fruit Crumble 111
- 148. Fruit Popsicles 112

STARRED DISHES 113
- 149. Beetroot carpaccio with rocket salad and walnuts 113
- 150. Saffron Risotto with Asparagus and Parmesan Shavings 114
- 151. Grilled Salmon with Ginger Lime Sauce 115
- 152. Saffron Risotto with Asparagus and Parmesan Shavings 116
- 153. Vegetable Flan with Light Cheese Fondue 117
- 154. Tuna Tartare with Guacamole 118
- 155. Soy Glazed Salmon with Ginger Lime Sauce and Crispy Salad 119
- 156. Chicken Breast Stuffed with Spinach and Ricotta with Mashed Potatoes and Sautéed Asparagus 120

CONCLUSION 121

AUTHOR INFORMATION

Chris Marshall is an author and researcher committed to promoting a healthy lifestyle through nutrition and physical activity. With a solid background and a passionate interest in nutrition and health, Chris devotes himself to studying and researching methods to counteract major health problems associated with poor diet.

Chris Marshall is dedicated to providing innovative, evidence-based approaches to addressing health challenges through diet and lifestyle. Through his research, he has developed effective strategies to restore proper bodily function, using nutrition as the foundation for well-being.

Chris Marshall's research focuses on the interconnections between diet and major diseases caused by an unhealthy lifestyle. Through in-depth studies and scientific analyses, Chris has identified how certain disorders, such as obesity, type 2 diabetes, cardiovascular diseases, and liver diseases, are closely linked to dietary habits and levels of physical activity.

Drawing on scientific foundations, Chris Marshall develops and recommends practical strategies to prevent and treat these diseases through changes in diet and lifestyle. His recommendations are designed to be realistic and sustainable in the long term, offering individuals effective tools to improve their health and reduce the risk of chronic diseases.

Follow Chris Marshall on Amazon to explore his publications and discover practical tips for improving your health through nutrition and physical activity.

BONUS 1

Fatty Liver

"Unlock the secrets of liver health! Scan the QR code and discover everything in our demonstrative video on fatty liver disease."

BONUS 2

Liver Cleanse Smoothies

"Scan the QR code and dive into a world of delicious and healthy smoothies! Get inspired to nourish your body and support your health with our recipe book of special smoothies for fatty liver disease."

BONUS 3

Gocery List

"Explore the convenience of a weekly grocery list for your liver health. Scan the QR code and access a comprehensive list of recommended foods instantly, making your shopping easier than ever."

BONUS 4

Meal Plane

"Create a health path for your fatty liver! Scan the QR code of the meal plan in our cookbook and start the journey towards a healthier life today."

BONUS 5

Fitness Liver

"Ready to transform your liver health? Scan the QR code and follow our specially designed workout plan for those with fatty liver disease."

BONUS 6

Fatty Liver Index

"Discover your liver steatosis index in an instant! Scan the QR code and take control of your health today."

Dear readers,

It is with great joy that we welcome you to this Liver Health Cookbook. First and foremost, we would like to express our sincere gratitude for choosing to purchase this book. We are excited to share with you a collection of recipes specifically designed for anyone interested in maintaining a healthy and balanced diet, especially those affected by fatty liver disease.

Fatty liver disease, a condition characterized by the accumulation of fat in the liver, requires special attention to diet. In this Cookbook, we have committed to providing tasty and nutritious dishes using affordable and readily available ingredients. Each recipe has been specially designed to offer a satisfying culinary experience without compromising liver health.

We hope that these recipes not only satisfy your palate but also inspire you to explore new ways to maintain a healthy and sustainable lifestyle. Your well-being is our priority, and we are excited to accompany you on this culinary journey.

Thank you again for your support and for choosing to take charge of your health with these tasty and healthy recipes.

INTRODUCTION

Fatty liver disease, commonly known as "fatty liver," is a condition characterized by the excessive accumulation of fat in liver cells. This accumulation can lead to a range of complications and health problems, making effective management of fatty liver disease a priority for many individuals.

Calculate Your Fatty Liver Index

The fatty liver index is a numerical score or evaluation system used to measure the severity or degree of fat accumulation in the liver. This index can be calculated using a combination of various clinical parameters, such as blood test results (triglycerides and GGT), body mass index (BMI). The fatty liver index can be useful for diagnosing and monitoring the condition of fatty liver and for assessing treatment response over time."

The liver is a vital organ responsible for a wide range of functions in the human body, including bile production, nutrient metabolism, detoxification of harmful substances, and regulation of blood sugar levels. When the liver is affected by fatty liver disease, its ability to perform these functions may be compromised, leading to a range of symptoms and complications.

Fatty liver disease can be divided into two main categories: non-alcoholic fatty liver disease (NAFLD) and alcoholic fatty liver disease (ALD). While ALD is caused by alcohol abuse, NAFLD is associated with factors such as obesity, type 2 diabetes, insulin resistance, and a sedentary lifestyle. NAFLD has become one of the most common liver diseases worldwide, with a significant impact on public health.

Diagnosis of fatty liver disease usually occurs through blood tests, liver ultrasounds, or liver biopsies. However, management of the condition primarily focuses on treating underlying risk factors and adopting a healthy lifestyle, including a balanced diet and regular exercise.

One of the key recommendations for managing fatty liver disease is adopting a nutrient-rich diet low in saturated fats and added sugars. This can help reduce the workload of the liver and improve its ability to metabolize excess fats. Some specific nutrients are particularly important for liver health, including lean proteins, fiber, omega-3 fatty acids, and antioxidants.

Additionally, it is essential to limit or avoid alcohol consumption, as it can contribute to fat accumulation in the liver and worsen the condition. Alcohol can also interfere with nutrient metabolism and damage liver cells, exacerbating the symptoms of fatty liver disease.

To learn more about the topic, click on the QR code below to watch a explanatory video.

In addition to diet, regular physical exercise is essential for improving liver health and reducing the risk of complications related to fatty liver disease. Physical activity helps burn excess fat, improve insulin sensitivity, and reduce inflammation in the body, all factors that can contribute to better management of the condition.

In the "Fatty Liver Cookbook," we are committed to providing a wide range of healthy and tasty recipes specifically designed to support liver health and manage fatty liver disease. Each recipe has been specially developed to be low in saturated fats and added sugars but rich in essential nutrients and delicious flavor. With our book, we hope to provide readers with the tools and resources needed to adopt a healthy lifestyle and successfully manage their fatty liver condition.

We hope you find inspiration and culinary delights within these pages. If you enjoy the recipes, we encourage you to share your experience by leaving a review. Bon appétit!

BREAKFAST

Sweet Breakfasts

1. Oat and Fruit Smoothie (Vegan)

 5 minutes

Nutritional Values (per serving): Calories: 250, Protein: 8g, Fat: 4g, Carbohydrates: 45g, Fiber: 7g, Sodium: 50mg

Ingredients (for one person):
- 1 ripe banana
- 1/2 cup strawberries
- 1/4 cup oats
- 1 cup unsweetened almond milk

Instructions:
1. Start by cutting the ripe banana into pieces.
2. Place the banana pieces and strawberries into the blender bowl.
3. Add oats and unsweetened almond milk.
4. Blend all the ingredients until smooth and homogeneous. If the mixture is too thick, you can add some water to reach the desired consistency.
5. Pour the smoothie into a glass and serve immediately to enjoy this delicious and nutritious morning beverage or refreshing snack! Enjoy!

2. Greek Yogurt with Honey and Almonds (Vegetarian)

 3 minutes

Nutritional Values (per serving): Calories: 200, Protein: 15g, Fat: 10g, Carbohydrates: 15g, Fiber: 2g, Sodium: 60mg

Ingredients (for one person):
- 1 cup Greek yogurt
- 1 tablespoon honey
- 1 handful of chopped almonds

Instructions:
1. Pour the Greek yogurt into a bowl.
2. Add honey to the yogurt.
3. Mix everything well until the honey is completely incorporated into the yogurt.
4. Sprinkle the surface of the yogurt with chopped almonds.
5. Serve immediately and enjoy this simple but delicious Greek yogurt with honey and almonds! Bon Appetit!

3. Quinoa Porridge with Fruit (Vegan)

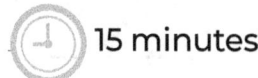 15 minutes

Nutritional Values (per serving): Calories: 300, Protein: 10g, Fat: 5g, Carbohydrates: 55g, Fiber: 6g, Sodium: 70mg

Ingredients (for one person):
- 1/4 cup quinoa
- 1/2 cup unsweetened coconut milk
- 1 sliced banana
- 1/4 cup fresh blueberries

Instructions:
1. Rinse the quinoa well under running water to remove any residues and starch.
2. In a saucepan, bring 1/2 cup of water to a boil and add the quinoa. Reduce the heat and let it simmer for about 12-15 minutes, or until the quinoa is tender and has absorbed the water.
3. Add the coconut milk to the cooked quinoa and mix well. Continue to cook for another 2-3 minutes until the porridge reaches the desired consistency.
4. Pour the quinoa porridge into a bowl and garnish with sliced bananas and fresh blueberries.
5. Serve the porridge hot and enjoy this nutritious and delicious breakfast! Bon Appetit!

4. Banana and Coconut Muffins (Vegetarian)

 25 minutes

Nutritional Values (per muffin): Calories: 180, Protein: 4g, Fat: 8g, Carbohydrates: 25g, Fiber: 3g, Sodium: 90mg

Ingredients (for one person):
- 1 ripe banana
- 1/4 cup sugar
- 1/4 cup coconut oil
- 1/4 egg
- 1/4 cup whole wheat flour
- 1/2 teaspoon baking powder

Instructions:
1. Preheat the oven to 180°C (350°F) and prepare a muffin tray with paper liners or lightly grease non-stick molds.
2. In a bowl, mash the banana with a fork until smooth.
3. Add sugar, coconut oil, and egg to the mashed banana. Mix well until homogeneous.
4. Incorporate the whole wheat flour and baking powder into the batter and gently mix until the dry ingredients are just incorporated. Be careful not to overmix to avoid developing too much gluten, which could make the muffins less fluffy.
5. Evenly distribute the batter into the muffin molds, filling each about 3/4 full.
6. Bake the muffins in the preheated oven for 15-20 minutes, or until the muffins are golden and a toothpick inserted into the center comes out clean.
7. Once baked, remove the muffins from the tray and let them cool on a wire rack for a few minutes before serving.
8. Your Banana and Coconut Muffins are ready! Enjoy them for breakfast or as a delicious snack.

Cocoa and Banana Pancakes (Vegetarian)

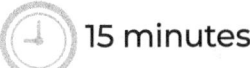 15 minutes

Nutritional Values (per serving): Calories: 250, Protein: 6g, Fat: 5g, Carbohydrates: 40g, Fiber: 4g, Sodium: 100mg

Ingredients (for one person):
- 1/2 ripe banana
- 1/4 cup whole wheat flour
- 1 tablespoon unsweetened cocoa powder
- 1/4 egg
- 1/4 cup unsweetened almond milk

Instructions:
1. Mash the banana in a bowl and mix it with the flour, cocoa powder, egg, and almond milk until you get a homogeneous mixture.
2. Lightly heat a non-stick skillet over medium heat.
3. Pour a ladleful of batter into the heated skillet and spread it evenly to form a pancake.
4. Cook the pancake for about 2-3 minutes until bubbles start to form on the surface and the edges become set.
5. Using a spatula, flip the pancake and cook for another 1-2 minutes until it is golden brown on both sides.
6. Repeat the process with the remaining batter.
7. Once all pancakes are cooked, serve them hot and garnish with fresh fruit, maple syrup, or yogurt as desired. Enjoy!

5. Cinnamon and Apple Muffins (Vegetarian)

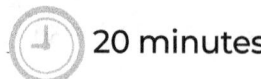 20 minutes

Nutritional Values (per muffin): Calories: 160, Protein: 3g, Fat: 5g, Carbohydrates: 30g, Fiber: 3g, Sodium: 90mg

Ingredients (for one person):

- 1/2 apple, diced
- 1 tablespoon sugar
- 1/4 egg
- 1/4 cup oil
- 1/4 cup whole wheat flour
- 1/2 teaspoon cinnamon

Instructions:

1. Preheat the oven to 180°C (350°F) and prepare a muffin tray with paper liners or lightly grease non-stick molds.
2. In a medium bowl, mix the diced apple with sugar until the apples are well coated with sugar.
3. Add the egg and oil to the sugared apples and mix well until homogeneous.
4. Add the whole wheat flour and cinnamon to the apple mixture and gently mix until the dry ingredients are just incorporated. Be careful not to overmix to avoid developing too much gluten, which could make the muffins less fluffy.
5. Evenly distribute the batter into the muffin molds, filling each about 3/4 full.
6. Bake the muffins in the preheated oven for 15-18 minutes, or until the muffins are golden and a toothpick inserted into the center comes out clean.
7. Once baked, remove the muffins from the tray and let them cool on a wire rack for a few minutes before serving.
8. Your delicious Cinnamon and Apple Muffins are ready to be enjoyed! Bon Appétit!

Savory Breakfasts

6. Scrambled Eggs with Spinach and Tomatoes (Vegetarian)

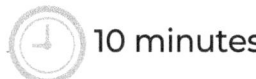 10 minutes

Nutritional Values (per serving): Calories: 220, Protein: 15g, Fat: 14g, Carbohydrates: 8g, Fiber: 3g, Sodium: 350mg

Ingredients (for one person):
- 2 eggs
- 1 cup fresh spinach, washed and chopped
- 1 medium tomato, diced
- Salt and pepper to taste
- Extra virgin olive oil

Instructions:
1. In a non-stick skillet, heat a drizzle of extra virgin olive oil over medium heat.
2. Add the chopped spinach and diced tomatoes to the skillet and cook for 2-3 minutes, stirring occasionally, until the spinach wilts and the tomatoes slightly soften.
3. Meanwhile, beat the eggs in a bowl and add a pinch of salt and pepper.
4. Pour the beaten eggs into the skillet with the spinach and tomatoes.
5. Cook the eggs, gently stirring with a spatula until they are cooked and well mixed with the spinach and tomatoes, about 2-3 minutes.
6. Once the eggs are cooked, transfer them to a serving plate and serve hot.
7. You can accompany the scrambled eggs with toast or a slice of whole wheat bread. Enjoy your meal!

7. Avocado and Egg Toast (Vegetarian)

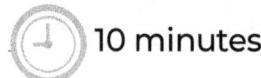 10 minutes

Nutritional Values (per serving): Calories: 300, Protein: 12g, Fat: 20g, Carbohydrates: 20g, Fiber: 8g, Sodium: 350mg

Ingredients (for one person):
- 1 slice of whole wheat bread
- 1 ripe avocado
- 1 egg
- Salt and pepper to taste
- Red pepper flakes (optional)
- Lemon juice (optional)

Instructions:
1. Toast the slice of whole wheat bread until crispy.
2. Meanwhile, cut the avocado in half, remove the pit, and scoop out the flesh with a spoon.
3. Mash the avocado in a bowl with a fork until creamy.
4. Add salt, pepper, and red pepper flakes (if desired) to the mashed avocado and mix well. You can also add a splash of lemon juice for a touch of freshness.
5. Heat a lightly greased non-stick skillet over medium heat.
6. Beat the egg and add it to the skillet, cooking until the yolk is done to your liking.
7. Spread the avocado mixture on the toasted bread slice and place the scrambled egg on top.
8. Finish with a sprinkle of freshly ground black pepper and, if desired, a few more red pepper flakes.
9. Serve the avocado and egg toast hot and enjoy immediately! Bon Appétit!

8. Spinach and Tomato Omelette (Vegetarian)

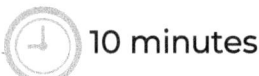 10 minutes

Nutritional Values (per serving): Calories: 250, Protein: 15g, Fat: 12g, Carbohydrates: 10g, Fiber: 3g, Sodium: 400mg

Ingredients (for one person):

- 2 eggs
- 1 handful of fresh spinach
- 1 medium tomato, diced
- Salt and pepper to taste
- Extra virgin olive oil

Instructions:

1. In a bowl, beat the eggs with a pinch of salt and pepper.
2. Heat a drizzle of extra virgin olive oil in a non-stick skillet over medium heat.
3. Add the fresh spinach to the skillet and cook for a couple of minutes until slightly wilted.
4. Add the diced tomato to the skillet with the spinach and stir for another minute.
5. Gently pour the beaten eggs into the skillet with the ingredients and spread them evenly.
6. Cook the omelette over medium-low heat until it begins to set around the edges.
7. Using a spatula, lift the edges of the omelette and tilt the skillet slightly to allow the liquid egg to flow onto the surface of the skillet. Repeat this process until the omelette is almost fully cooked.
8. Once the omelette is cooked underneath but still slightly soft on top, fold it in half with the help of the spatula.
9. Transfer the omelette to a serving plate and serve hot.
10. 1You can accompany the omelette with a slice of toast or a mixed salad for a complete meal. Enjoy your meal!

9. Sweet Potato Pancakes (Vegetarian)

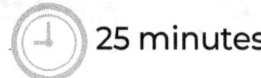 25 minutes

Nutritional Values (per serving): Calories: 220, Protein: 5g, Fat: 2g, Carbohydrates: 45g, Fiber: 5g, Sodium: 300mg

Ingredients (for one person):

- 1 small sweet potato
- 1 egg
- 2 tablespoons flour
- 1/2 teaspoon baking powder
- 1/4 teaspoon ground cinnamon
- Pinch of salt
- Olive oil (for cooking)

Instructions:

1. Preheat a non-stick skillet over medium-low heat.
2. Peel the sweet potato and finely grate it using a coarse grater.
3. Squeeze the grated sweet potato between your hands to remove excess moisture.
4. In a bowl, beat the egg and add the grated sweet potato.
5. Add the flour, baking powder, cinnamon, and salt. Mix well until you get a smooth batter.
6. Add a drizzle of olive oil to the hot skillet.
7. Pour a ladleful of pancake batter into the skillet and spread it evenly with the back of the spoon.
8. Cook the pancake for about 2-3 minutes per side, or until it becomes golden and crispy.
9. Repeat the process with the remaining batter.
10. 1Once cooked, serve the sweet potato pancakes hot and garnish them as desired with maple syrup, fresh fruit, or Greek yogurt. Enjoy your meal!

10. Buckwheat Pancakes with Yogurt and Fresh Fruit (Vegetarian)

⏲ 20 minutes

Nutritional Values (per serving): Calories: 280, Protein: 10g, Fat: 7g, Carbohydrates: 45g, Fiber: 6g, Sodium: 180mg

Ingredients (for one person):

- 1/2 cup buckwheat flour
- 1 egg
- 1/2 cup milk
- 1 tablespoon olive oil
- 1 teaspoon honey
- 1/2 teaspoon baking powder
- Pinch of salt
- Greek yogurt
- Fresh fruit of choice (strawberries, bananas, blueberries, etc.)

Instructions:

1. In a bowl, mix the buckwheat flour, baking powder, and salt.
2. In another bowl, beat the egg and add the milk, olive oil, and honey. Mix the liquid ingredients well.
3. Gradually pour the liquid ingredients into the bowl of dry ingredients, stirring until you get a smooth batter.
4. Heat a non-stick skillet over medium heat and lightly grease it with olive oil.
5. Pour a ladleful of pancake batter into the hot skillet and cook until bubbles form on the surface (about 2-3 minutes).
6. Flip the pancake and cook on the other side for another 1-2 minutes, or until golden.
7. Repeat the process with the remaining batter.
8. Once cooked, serve the pancakes on a plate and garnish with Greek yogurt and fresh fruit of your choice.
9. Add a drizzle of honey or maple syrup if you desire an extra touch of sweetness.
10. 1Serve the pancakes hot and enjoy them for breakfast or as a healthy snack. Bon Appétit!

11. Chickpea Cream and Tomato Toast (Vegetarian)

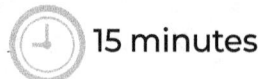 15 minutes

Nutritional Values (per serving): Calories: 280, Protein: 10g, Fat: 8g, Carbohydrates: 40g, Fiber: 8g, Sodium: 320mg

Ingredients (for one person):
- 2 slices of whole wheat bread
- 1/2 cup cooked chickpeas
- 1 clove garlic, minced
- Juice of 1/2 lemon
- Salt and pepper to taste
- Cherry tomatoes, halved
- Fresh basil leaves
- Extra virgin olive oil

Instructions:
1. In a small bowl, mash the cooked chickpeas with a potato masher or fork until creamy.
2. Add the minced garlic clove and lemon juice to the chickpea cream. Mix well and adjust salt and pepper to taste.
3. Toast the slices of whole wheat bread.
4. Spread the chickpea cream generously on the toasted bread slices.
5. Arrange the halved cherry tomatoes on top of the chickpea cream.
6. Place a few fresh basil leaves over the tomatoes.
7. Drizzle some extra virgin

Meat-Based Dishes

12. Chicken Curry with Brown Rice

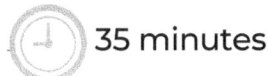 35 minutes

Nutritions: Calories: 320, Protein: 23g, Fat: 10g, Carbohydrates: 30g, Fiber: 4g, Sodium: 340mg

Ingredients:
- 2 chicken breasts, diced
- 1 cup coconut milk
- 1 cup diced tomatoes
- 1 onion, finely chopped
- 2 cloves garlic, minced
- 2 tablespoons curry paste
- 1 cup brown rice
- Salt to taste
- Black pepper to taste
- Olive oil

Instructions:
1. Heat a drizzle of olive oil in a large non-stick skillet over medium-high heat.
2. Add the chopped onions and minced garlic to the skillet and sauté until they become translucent and slightly golden.
3. Add the diced chicken breasts to the skillet and cook until they are golden brown on all sides.
4. Once the chicken is browned, add the diced tomatoes and curry paste to the skillet. Mix well to evenly distribute the curry paste.
5. Pour the coconut milk into the skillet and bring it to a boil. Reduce the heat and let it simmer for about 15-20 minutes, or until the chicken is fully cooked and the sauce has slightly thickened.
6. Meanwhile, cook the brown rice according to the instructions on the package.
7. Once the chicken curry is ready and the rice is cooked to your desired consistency, serve it hot over a bed of steamed brown rice.
8. Adjust salt and pepper to taste and garnish with fresh coriander leaves if desired.

13. Turkey Meatloaf with Mashed Potatoes and Carrots

Ingredients:
- 125g ground turkey
- 1/4 onion, finely chopped
- 1 clove garlic, minced
- 1 tablespoon fresh parsley, chopped
- 1/4 cup whole wheat breadcrumbs
- 1 medium potato, peeled and diced
- 1 medium carrot, peeled and sliced
- Salt to taste
- Black pepper to taste
- Olive oil

Instructions:
1. Preheat the oven to 180°C and line a small baking sheet with parchment paper.
2. In a small bowl, mix the ground turkey with the chopped onion, minced garlic, chopped fresh parsley, and whole wheat breadcrumbs. Season with salt and pepper to taste.
3. Once the ingredients are well combined, transfer the mixture onto a clean work surface and shape it into a small, compact round meatloaf.
4. Place the meatloaf on the prepared baking sheet and bake in the preheated oven for about 20-25 minutes, or until the meatloaf is golden brown and fully cooked.
5. Meanwhile, bring a pot of water to a boil and add the diced potatoes and sliced carrots. Cook until the vegetables are tender, about 10-15 minutes.
6. Drain the potatoes and carrots and transfer them to a small bowl. Add a pinch of salt and pepper and mash the vegetables until smooth and creamy.
7. Once cooked, remove the turkey meatloaf from the oven and let it rest for a few minutes before serving.
8. Serve the sliced meatloaf with the warm mashed potatoes and carrots. Enjoy!

14. Chicken alla Pizzaiola with Brown Rice

🕐 35 minutes

Nutritions: Calories: 320, Protein: 25g, Fat: 12g, Carbohydrates: 30g, Fiber: 4g, Sodium: 350mg

Ingredients:
- 2 chicken breasts
- 2 cups diced tomatoes
- 2 cloves garlic, minced
- 1 teaspoon dried oregano
- 1 teaspoon dried basil
- Salt to taste
- Black pepper to taste
- Olive oil
- 1 cup brown rice

Instructions:
1. Begin by cooking the brown rice. Rinse it under running water and place it in a pot with double the amount of water. Bring to a boil, then reduce the heat and let it cook covered for about 30 minutes, or until the rice is cooked and the water has been absorbed. Set aside.
2. Meanwhile, heat some olive oil in a non-stick skillet over medium-high heat. Add the chicken breasts and cook them for 5-6 minutes per side, or until they are golden brown and fully cooked. Remove the chicken from the skillet and set aside.
3. In the same skillet, add the minced garlic cloves and cook for a couple of minutes until they are golden and fragrant.
4. Add the diced tomatoes, dried oregano, and dried basil to the skillet. Mix well and let it cook for another 5-7 minutes, or until the tomatoes have slightly softened and released their juices.
5. Adjust salt and pepper according to your taste.
6. Add the cooked chicken breasts back to the skillet with the tomato sauce, making sure to coat them well with the sauce. Cook for another 2-3 minutes to allow the flavors to meld.
7. Arrange the steamed brown rice on serving plates and place the chicken breasts with the tomato sauce on top
8. Serve hot and garnish with fresh basil or chopped parsley if desired. Enjoy!

15. Quinoa Salad with Grilled Chicken

 30 minutes

Nutritions: Calories: 320, Protein: 25g, Fat: 12g, Carbohydrates: 28g, Fiber: 6g, Sodium: 280mg

Ingredients:
- 1 cup quinoa
- 1 bell pepper, diced
- 1 cucumber, diced
- 1 cup cherry tomatoes, halved
- 1/2 red onion, diced
- 2 chicken breasts, grilled and chopped
- Juice of 1 lemon
- 2 tablespoons chopped fresh herbs (parsley, basil, chives, etc.)
- Salt to taste
- Black pepper to taste
- Extra virgin olive oil

Instructions:
1. Begin by cooking the quinoa. Rinse it under cold water and place it in a pot with double the amount of water. Bring to a boil, then reduce the heat, cover, and let it simmer for about 15 minutes, or until all the water is absorbed. Once cooked, transfer it to a large bowl and let it cool slightly.
2. Add the diced bell pepper, cucumber, halved cherry tomatoes, and diced red onion to the bowl with the quinoa.
3. Add the grilled chicken pieces to the bowl with the other ingredients.
4. Prepare the dressing by mixing lemon juice, chopped fresh herbs, salt, and pepper in a small bowl. Pour the dressing over the quinoa and other ingredients in the bowl and mix well to distribute it evenly.
5. Taste and adjust salt and pepper according to your personal preference.
6. Transfer the quinoa and dressing to a serving platter and serve immediately as a delicious and nutritious one-dish meal.

16. Couscous with Chicken Curry

 25 minutes

Nutritions: Calories: 310, Protein: 20g, Fat: 10g, Carbohydrates: 30g, Fiber: 4g, Sodium: 280mg

Ingredients:

- 1 cup couscous
- 2 chicken breasts, cubed
- 2 tablespoons olive oil
- 1 onion, chopped
- 2 cloves garlic, minced
- 1 teaspoon curry powder
- 1/2 teaspoon turmeric powder
- 1/2 teaspoon chili powder (optional, for a spicy kick)
- 1 cup peas, fresh or frozen
- 1 carrot, thinly sliced
- 1 bell pepper, sliced
- Salt and pepper to taste
- Fresh parsley, chopped (for garnish)

Instructions:

- Prepare the Couscous:
1. In a pot, bring 1 cup of slightly salted water to a boil.
2. Place the couscous in a bowl and pour the boiling water over it.
3. Cover with a lid and let it sit for about 5-10 minutes, until the couscous has absorbed all the liquid and is fluffy.
4. Fluff the couscous with a fork to make it airy.
   - Prepare the Chicken Curry:
5. In a large skillet, heat the olive oil over medium heat.
6. Add the chopped onion and minced garlic and sauté until golden and soft.
7. Add the cubed chicken breasts and cook until golden brown on all sides, ensuring they are fully cooked.
8. Add the curry powder, turmeric, and chili powder (if using), stirring well to evenly coat the chicken with the spices.
9. Add the peas, sliced carrots, and bell pepper to the skillet and mix well.
10. Cover the skillet and cook over medium-low heat for about 8-10 minutes, stirring occasionally, until the vegetables are tender and the chicken is fully cooked.
11. Ensure that the curry sauce is reduced and thickened.
    - Serve:
12. Arrange the couscous on a serving plate and pour the chicken curry and vegetables over it.
13. Garnish with chopped fresh parsley.
14. Serve hot and enjoy!
15. This delicious and nutritious recipe is perfect for a complete and satisfying meal, offering a mix of proteins, carbohydrates, and vegetables, ideal for a balanced diet. Enjoy!

17. Whole Wheat Tagliatelle with Turkey and Mushroom Sauce

Nutritions: Calories: Approximately 360 kcal, Protein: Approximately 22g, Fat: Approximately 13g, Carbohydrates: Approximately 38g, Fiber: Approximately 5g, Sodium: Approximately 300mg

Ingredients:

- 60g whole wheat tagliatelle
- 75g lean ground turkey
- 50g fresh mushrooms (porcini, button mushrooms, or mixed mushrooms)
- 1/2 medium onion, finely chopped
- 1 clove garlic, minced
- 50g diced tomatoes (fresh or canned)
- 1 tablespoon olive oil
- Salt and pepper to taste
- Fresh parsley, chopped (for garnish)

Instructions:

- Prepare the Tagliatelle:
1. In a large pot, bring a generous amount of salted water to a boil.
2. Add the whole wheat tagliatelle and cook according to the package instructions until al dente.
3. Drain the tagliatelle and set aside.
- Prepare the Turkey and Mushroom Sauce:
4. In a non-stick skillet, heat the olive oil over medium heat.
5. Add the chopped onion and garlic and sauté until golden and soft.
6. Add the lean ground turkey and cook, breaking up any clumps with a wooden spoon, until fully browned and cooked through.
7. Add the sliced fresh mushrooms and cook until they are soft and have released their juices.
8. Add the diced tomatoes and mix well. Cook for a few minutes until the tomatoes have slightly thickened.
9. Season with salt and pepper to taste.
- Complete the Dish:
10. Pour the cooked whole wheat tagliatelle into the skillet with the turkey and mushroom sauce and mix well to combine all the ingredients.
11. Cook over medium-low heat for a few minutes, stirring occasionally, to allow the flavors to meld.
12. Once the tagliatelle is well coated with the sauce, turn off the heat.
13. Serve the whole wheat tagliatelle with turkey and mushroom sauce on a plate, garnishing with a sprinkle of chopped fresh parsley.

18. Lemon Chicken with Grilled Asparagus

Nutritional Information (per serving): Calories: Approximately 300, Protein: 30g, Fat: 10g, Carbohydrates: 10g, Fiber: 3g, Sodium: 250mg

Ingredients:
- 2 chicken breasts, thinly sliced
- Juice of 1 lemon
- 2 cloves garlic, minced
- Black pepper to taste
- Fresh parsley, chopped
- 1 bunch of asparagus
- Salt to taste
- Extra virgin olive oil

Instructions:
1. In a bowl, mix lemon juice, minced garlic, black pepper, and fresh parsley. Add the chicken breast slices to the marinade, ensuring they are completely coated. Cover the bowl and let it marinate in the refrigerator for at least 15-20 minutes.
2. Heat a non-stick skillet over medium-high heat. Once hot, add the marinated chicken slices and cook for about 5-7 minutes per side, or until the chicken is fully cooked and has achieved a uniform golden brown color. Ensure the chicken is cooked through but not dry.
3. Meanwhile, prepare the asparagus. Trim off the woody ends and wash them under running water. Heat a grill or grill pan and brush the asparagus with a drizzle of olive oil. Grill the asparagus for about 5-7 minutes, turning occasionally, until tender but still crisp.
4. Arrange the grilled chicken and asparagus on a serving platter. Season with salt and pepper if needed.
5. Serve immediately as a light and flavorful main dish.

19. Turkey Taco Bowl with Brown Rice

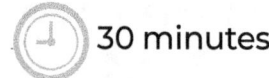 30 minutes

Nutritional Information (per serving): Calories: 330 kcal, Protein: 20g, Fat: 15g, Carbohydrates: 28g, Fiber: 6g, Sodium: 360mg

Ingredients:

- 125g ground turkey
- 1/2 teaspoon taco seasoning mix
- 1/2 cup cooked brown rice
- 1/4 cup black beans, rinsed and drained
- 1/4 cup corn
- 1/2 ripe avocado, diced
- Fresh tomato salsa (pico de gallo or similar)
- Salt and pepper to taste
- Fresh cilantro (optional), chopped

Instructions:

1. In a non-stick skillet, cook the ground turkey over medium-high heat until fully cooked and beginning to brown. Add the taco seasoning mix and stir well, ensuring it is evenly distributed. Continue to cook for a few minutes for the flavors to meld. Season with salt and pepper if needed.
2. While the turkey is cooking, heat the black beans and corn in a separate pot or in the microwave.
3. To prepare the brown rice, follow the package instructions for cooking. Be sure to rinse the rice well before cooking to remove excess starch.
4. Once cooked, place the brown rice at the bottom of a bowl. Top with the seasoned ground turkey, black beans, and corn.
5. Garnish the taco bowl with fresh diced avocado and fresh tomato salsa.
6. If desired, sprinkle with chopped fresh cilantro for an extra touch of freshness.
7. Serve immediately, mixing all the ingredients together before enjoying this delicious and nutritious taco bowl.

20. Beef Stew with Vegetables:

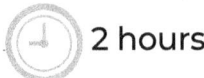 2 hours

Nutritional Information (per serving):: Calories: Approximately 300 kcal, Protein: Approximately 25-30g, Fat: Approximately 10-12g, Carbohydrates: Approximately 15-20g, Fiber: Approximately 4-6g, Sodium: Approximately 300mg

Ingredients:
- 150g lean beef, cubed
- 1 carrot, diced
- 1 stalk celery, diced
- 1/2 onion, chopped
- 250ml low-sodium vegetable broth
- 1/2 tablespoon olive oil (optional)
- Salt and pepper to taste
- Fresh parsley, chopped (for garnish)

Instructions:
1. Prepare the Ingredients:
   - Cut the lean beef into cubes and prepare the vegetables as instructed.
2. Cook the Stew:
   - In a large pot, heat the vegetable broth over medium-low heat.
   - If desired, you can add a little olive oil to sauté the vegetables, but it's optional.
   - Add the cubed beef to the pot and lightly brown it on all sides.
   - Add the diced carrot, celery, and chopped onion to the pot with the beef and mix well.
   - Pour the hot vegetable broth over the meat and vegetables, ensuring they are completely covered by the liquid.
   - Bring everything to a boil, then reduce the heat to low and let it simmer for about 1.5 2 hours, or until the meat is tender and the vegetables are well-cooked.
   - During cooking, if necessary, add some hot water to prevent the broth from drying out too much.
   - Taste the stew and adjust the seasoning with salt and pepper, if necessary.
3. Serving:
   - Once the stew is ready, turn off the heat and let it rest for a few minutes.
   - Serve the hot beef stew in a bowl, garnishing with chopped fresh parsley, if desired.

21. Lean Beef Chili

 15 minutes 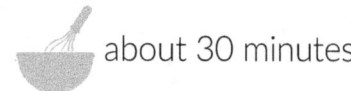 about 30 minutes

Nutritional Values (per approximate serving): Calories: about 280 kcal, Protein: variable, about 15-20g, Fat: variable, about 5-10g, Carbohydrates: variable, about 30-40g, Fiber: about 6g, Sodium: about 320mg

Ingredients:
- 150g lean ground beef
- 1/2 onion, chopped
- 1/2 bell pepper, diced
- 200g diced tomatoes (canned or fresh)
- 200g canned red kidney beans, rinsed and drained
- 200g canned black beans, rinsed and drained
- 1/2 cup corn (canned or fresh)
- 1 cup vegetable broth
- 1 teaspoon chili powder
- 1/2 teaspoon ground cumin
- 1/2 teaspoon paprika
- Salt and pepper to taste
- Fresh cilantro (optional), chopped, for garnish

Instructions:
1. In a large pot, heat a little oil over medium heat. Add the lean ground beef and cook until browned and fully cooked, breaking it up with a spatula to avoid clumps. Remove any excess fat.
2. Add the chopped onion and diced bell pepper to the pot and cook for about 5 minutes, or until the vegetables are soft.
3. Add the diced tomatoes, drained red kidney beans, drained black beans, and corn to the pot. Mix the ingredients well.
4. Pour the vegetable broth into the pot and season with chili powder, ground cumin, and paprika. Mix everything well.
5. Bring the chili to a boil, then reduce the heat and let it simmer for about 30 minutes, stirring occasionally. Make sure the chili is hot and the ingredients are well combined.
6. Taste and adjust seasoning with salt and pepper if necessary. If desired, you can add more spices to enhance the flavor.
7. Serve the hot chili, garnished with chopped fresh cilantro if desired. Serve with toasted bread or brown rice, if preferred.

22. Turkey and Black Bean Chili

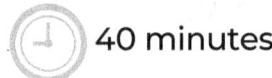 40 minutes

Nutritional Values (per serving): Calories: about 310 kcal, Carbohydrates: about 25g, Protein: about 23g, Fat: about 9g, Fiber: 6g, Sodium: 260mg

Ingredients:

- 150g ground turkey
- 1/4 onion, chopped
- 1/2 teaspoon chili powder
- 1/2 teaspoon ground cumin
- 200g diced tomatoes (canned or fresh)
- 1/2 green bell pepper, diced
- 100g canned black beans, rinsed and drained
- 1/2 cup vegetable broth
- Fresh cilantro, chopped, for garnish
- Lime wedges, for serving

Instructions:

1. In a large pot, heat a little olive oil over medium heat. Add the ground turkey and cook until browned and fully cooked, breaking it up with a spatula to avoid clumps.
2. Add the chopped onion, chili powder, and ground cumin to the pot with the turkey and cook for about 5 minutes, or until the onion is soft.
3. Add the diced tomatoes, green bell pepper, drained black beans, and vegetable broth to the pot. Mix the ingredients well.
4. Bring the chili to a boil, then reduce the heat and let it simmer for about 30 minutes, stirring occasionally. Make sure the chili is hot and the ingredients are well combined.
5. Taste and adjust seasoning with salt and pepper if necessary.
6. Serve the hot chili, garnished with chopped fresh cilantro and a lime wedge on each portion.

23. Baked Chicken Meatballs with Sweet Potatoes

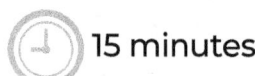 15 minutes   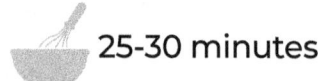 25-30 minutes

Nutritional Values (per serving): Calories: about 300 kcal, Protein: about 20-25g, Fat: about 10-15g, Carbohydrates: about 30-35g, Fiber: about 4g, Sodium: about 270mg

Ingredients:
- 125g ground chicken
- 1/4 onion, chopped
- 1/2 tablespoon fresh parsley, chopped
- 1 tablespoon whole wheat breadcrumbs
- Salt and pepper to taste
- Olive oil
- 1/2 sweet potato, sliced
- Assorted vegetables (such as zucchini, carrots, bell peppers)

Instructions:
1. **Preparation:** Preheat the oven to 200°C (400°F) and line a baking sheet with parchment paper. Slice the sweet potato and prepare the assorted vegetables.
2. **Preparing the Meatballs:** In a bowl, mix together the ground chicken, chopped onion, fresh parsley, and whole wheat breadcrumbs. Add salt and pepper to taste and form uniform-sized meatballs. Place them on the prepared baking sheet.
3. **Preparing the Sweet Potatoes:** Arrange the sweet potato slices on another baking sheet. Drizzle with olive oil, salt, and pepper.
4. **Baking:** Place both baking sheets in the preheated oven and bake for 25-30 minutes, or until the meatballs are golden and cooked through, and the sweet potatoes are soft and slightly crispy.
5. **Preparing the Vegetables:** While the meatballs and sweet potatoes bake, prepare the assorted vegetables by cutting them into pieces and seasoning with olive oil, salt, and pepper.
6. **Serving:** Once cooked, remove the chicken meatballs and sweet potatoes from the oven. Serve them hot with the assorted vegetables as a side dish. Enjoy your meal!

24. Veal Steak with Arugula and Tomato Salad

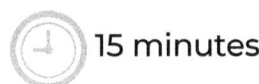 15 minutes   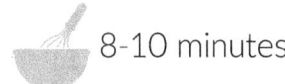 8-10 minutes

Nutritional Values (per approximate serving): Calories: about 290, Protein: about 25-30g, Fat: about 15-20g, Carbohydrates: about 5-10g, Fiber: about 3g, Sodium: about 260mg

Ingredients:
- 1 slice of veal steak (about 150g)
- 1 sprig of fresh rosemary
- 1 clove of garlic, minced
- A handful of fresh arugula
- 4-5 cherry tomatoes, halved
- 1 teaspoon reduced balsamic vinegar
- 1 teaspoon extra virgin olive oil
- Salt and pepper to taste

Instructions:
1. Preheat the grill to medium-high heat.
2. Marinate the veal steak with fresh rosemary, minced garlic, salt, and pepper for about 10 minutes.
3. Grill the marinated veal steak for about 4-5 minutes per side, or until cooked to perfection.
4. Meanwhile, prepare the salad: in a bowl, mix the fresh arugula and halved cherry tomatoes.
5. Dress the salad with reduced balsamic vinegar and extra virgin olive oil, and gently toss.
6. Once cooked, transfer the veal steak to a cutting board and let it rest for a few minutes.
7. Slice the meat thinly against the grain.
8. Arrange the meat slices on top of the arugula and tomato salad.
9. Finish the dish with a light drizzle of reduced balsamic vinegar and a drizzle of extra virgin olive oil. Serve immediately. Enjoy your meal!

Fish-Based Dishes

25. Grilled Salmon with Lemon and Caper Sauce

 20 minutes   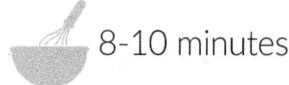 8-10 minutes

Nutritional Values (per approximate serving): Calories: about 300, Protein: 25g, Fat: 18g, Carbohydrates: 2g, Fiber: 2g, Sodium: 250mg

Ingredients:
- 1 salmon fillet
- Juice of 1 lemon
- 1 tablespoon capers, chopped
- 1 tablespoon fresh parsley, chopped
- Salt and pepper to taste

Instructions:
1. Preheat the grill to medium-high heat.
2. Season the salmon fillet with fresh lemon juice, chopped capers, fresh parsley, salt, and pepper.
3. Place the seasoned salmon fillet on the preheated grill.
4. Grill the salmon for about 4-5 minutes per side, or until cooked evenly and flakes easily with a fork.
5. Once cooked, remove the salmon from the grill and transfer it to a serving plate.
6. Finish the dish with a generous drizzle of additional lemon juice.
7. Serve the grilled salmon with lemon and caper sauce hot and accompany it with your choice of side dishes. Enjoy your meal!

26. Steamed Salmon with Zucchini Risotto

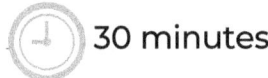 30 minutes

Nutritions: Calories: about 320 per serving, Protein: 25g, Fat: 12g, Carbohydrates: 30g, Fiber: 4g, Sodium: 280mg

Ingredients:
- 4 salmon fillets
- 2 zucchinis, diced
- 1 cup brown rice
- Bay leaves
- Chopped fresh parsley
- Grated lemon zest
- Salt and pepper to taste

Instructions:
1. Cook the brown rice according to package instructions.
2. Meanwhile, cut the salmon into cubes and place it in a steaming basket. Add some bay leaves to the salmon for flavoring.
3. Steam the salmon for about 8-10 minutes or until cooked and tender.
4. Once the rice is cooked, transfer it to a bowl and add the diced zucchinis, chopped fresh parsley, and grated lemon zest. Mix well to incorporate the ingredients.
5. Arrange the zucchini risotto on serving plates and place the steamed salmon cubes on top of the risotto.
6. Finish the dish with a squeeze of fresh lemon juice, if desired, and serve hot. Enjoy!

27. Tuna and Orzo Salad

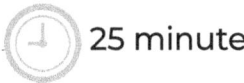 25 minutes

Nutritions: Calories: about 280 per serving, Protein: 20g, Fat: 8g, Carbohydrates: 35g, Fiber: 5g, Sodium: 290mg

Ingredients:
- 1 cup orzo
- 1 can tuna, drained
- 1 cup cherry tomatoes, halved
- 1 cucumber, diced
- 1/4 cup pitted black olives, sliced
- Chopped fresh basil
- Olive oil
- White wine vinegar
- Salt and pepper

Instructions:
1. Cook the orzo in salted boiling water according to package instructions. Once cooked, drain and let it cool.
2. In a large bowl, mix the cooked orzo with the drained tuna, halved cherry tomatoes, diced cucumber, sliced black olives, and chopped fresh basil.
3. Dress the salad with olive oil and white wine vinegar, then season with salt and pepper to taste.
4. Mix all the ingredients well to evenly distribute the dressing.
5. Serve the tuna and orzo salad as a light and nutritious main dish. Enjoy your meal!

28. Tuna and Tomato Pasta Salad

Nutritional Values (per serving): Calories: about 300, Protein: 15g, Fat: 10g, Carbohydrates: 40g, Fiber: 4g, Sodium: 280mg

Ingredients:
- 100g short pasta (penne, fusilli, farfalle, etc.)
- 1/2 can of canned tuna, drained
- 1/2 cup cherry tomatoes, halved
- 2 tablespoons pitted black olives
- Chopped fresh basil, to taste
- Lemon juice, to taste
- 1 tablespoon olive oil
- Salt and pepper, to taste

Instructions:
1. Preparing the Pasta:
   - Cook the pasta in a large pot of salted boiling water according to package instructions. Once cooked, drain it and let it cool slightly.
2. Preparing the Salad:
   - In a large bowl, combine the cooked pasta, drained tuna, halved cherry tomatoes, and pitted black olives.
   - Add chopped fresh basil to flavor the salad.
3. Dressing:
   - Add a drizzle of lemon juice to freshen up the salad.
   - Pour olive oil and mix well to evenly distribute the dressing.
   - Adjust salt and pepper according to your taste.
4. Serving:
   - Transfer the tuna and tomato pasta salad to a serving platter.
   - Serve immediately as a light and tasty main dish.
   - This pasta salad is perfect for a refreshing and flavorful meal, rich in protein and carbohydrates. Enjoy your meal!

29. Salmon Meatballs with Brown Rice and Grilled Vegetables

 35 minutes 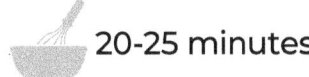 20-25 minutes

Nutritional Values (per serving): Calories: about 320, Protein: 22g, Fat: 12g, Carbohydrates: 30g, Fiber: 5g, Sodium: 290mg

Ingredients:

- 150g salmon fillet, minced
- 1/4 cup whole wheat breadcrumbs
- 1/2 egg (lightly beaten, use half)
- 1 tablespoon chopped fresh parsley
- 1/2 teaspoon garlic powder
- Ground black pepper, to taste
- 1/2 cup brown rice
- Mixed vegetables for grilling (zucchini, bell peppers, eggplant)
- Olive oil, as needed
- Salt, as needed

Instructions:

1. In a large bowl, mix minced salmon with whole wheat breadcrumbs, half beaten egg, chopped fresh parsley, garlic powder, and ground black pepper. Ensure the ingredients are well combined.
2. Shape the mixture into meatballs, compacting them well so they don't fall apart during cooking.
3. In a lightly oiled non-stick skillet, cook the salmon meatballs over medium-high heat until they are golden brown on all sides and fully cooked through, about 10-12 minutes.
4. Meanwhile, cook the brown rice according to package instructions.
5. Cut the selected vegetables (zucchini, bell peppers, eggplant) into slices or pieces, then grill them on a grill or grill pan for about 5-7 minutes, or until tender and slightly charred.
6. Once cooked, serve the salmon meatballs with cooked brown rice and grilled vegetables as a side. Adjust salt and pepper to taste. Enjoy your meal!

30. Lemon Shrimp Risotto

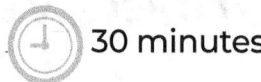 30 minutes

Nutritions: Calories: about 330 per serving, Protein: 20g, Fat: 8g, Carbohydrates: 40g, Fiber: 3g, Sodium: 290mg

Ingredients:

- 1 cup brown rice
- 2 cups vegetable broth
- Zest of 1 lemon
- Juice of 1 lemon
- 200g peeled shrimp
- Chopped fresh parsley, as needed
- Salt, as needed
- Ground black pepper, as needed

Instructions:

1. In a saucepan, bring the vegetable broth to a boil, then reduce the heat and keep it warm over low heat.
2. In a non-stick skillet, toast the brown rice dry for about 2-3 minutes, stirring occasionally, until it becomes slightly golden and fragrant.
3. Add a ladleful of warm broth to the toasted rice and stir continuously until the broth is absorbed. Continue adding the broth one ladle at a time, stirring occasionally, until the rice is al dente and has absorbed almost all the broth, about 20-25 minutes.
4. Add the grated lemon zest and lemon juice to the risotto, mix well, and cook for another 2-3 minutes.
5. Meanwhile, in a separate pan, cook the peeled shrimp with a drizzle of olive oil until they are pink and cooked through, about 3-4 minutes.
6. Once the rice is cooked and the desired consistency is achieved, adjust salt and pepper to taste.
7. Serve the lemon risotto on serving plates and garnish with cooked shrimp and a generous sprinkle of chopped fresh parsley. Enjoy your meal!

31. Couscous Salad with Smoked Salmon

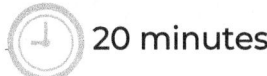 20 minutes

Nutritions: Calories: about 310 per serving, Protein: about 15g, Fat: about 10g, Carbohydrates: about 35g, Fiber: 5g, Sodium: 280mg

Ingredients:
- 1 cup couscous
- 100g smoked salmon, thinly sliced
- 1/2 cup canned chickpeas, drained and rinsed
- 1/2 cup cherry tomatoes, halved
- 1/4 cup pickled cucumbers
- Chopped fresh parsley, to taste
- Olive oil, to taste
- Lemon juice, to taste
- Salt, to taste
- Black pepper, to taste

Instructions:
1. Prepare the couscous according to the package instructions and let it cool.
2. In a large bowl, mix the cooled couscous with the thinly sliced smoked salmon, drained and rinsed chickpeas, halved cherry tomatoes, and pickled cucumbers.
3. Dress the salad with a drizzle of olive oil, freshly squeezed lemon juice, chopped fresh parsley, salt, and freshly ground black pepper to taste.
4. Mix all the ingredients well until evenly distributed and well seasoned.
5. Serve the couscous salad with smoked salmon as a light and flavorful side dish or as a main course for a healthy and satisfying meal. Enjoy your meal!

32. Shrimp and Pineapple Skewers with Brown Rice

 25 minutes

Nutritional Values (per serving): Calories: about 310 kcal, Protein: about 20g, Fat: about 5g, Carbohydrates: about 50g, Fiber: about 4g, Sodium: about 280mg

Ingredients:

- 100g raw shrimp, peeled and cleaned
- 100g fresh pineapple, cut into cubes
- 50g brown rice
- Mixed vegetables for stir-frying (of your choice, about 100g)

Instructions:

1. Preheat the grill to medium-high heat.
2. Prepare the skewers by alternating raw shrimp and pineapple cubes on skewers. If necessary, use 2-3 shrimp and pieces of pineapple per skewer.
3. Lightly brush the skewers with some olive oil to prevent sticking to the grill.
4. Grill the skewers for about 2-3 minutes per side, or until the shrimp are pink and fully cooked.
5. Meanwhile, cook the brown rice according to the package instructions.
6. In a non-stick skillet, stir-fry the mixed vegetables with a drizzle of olive oil until they are tender but still crisp.
7. Serve the hot shrimp and pineapple skewers alongside the cooked brown rice and stir-fried vegetables. Enjoy your meal!

33. Salmon with Almond Crust and Steamed Broccoli

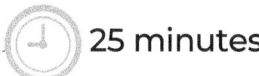 25 minutes

Nutritions: Calories: about 290 per serving, Protein: about 25g, Fat: about 15g, Carbohydrates: about 8g, Fiber: 4g, Sodium: 260mg

Ingredients:
- Salmon fillets
- Ground almonds
- Chopped fresh parsley
- Grated lemon zest
- Fresh broccoli
- Lemon juice

Instructions:
1. Preheat the oven to 200°C and line a baking sheet with parchment paper.
2. In a bowl, mix ground almonds, chopped fresh parsley, and grated lemon zest.
3. Place the salmon fillets on the prepared baking sheet and evenly coat them with the almond mixture.
4. Bake the salmon for about 15-20 minutes, or until cooked through and the almond crust is golden and crispy.
5. Meanwhile, steam the broccoli until tender but still crisp.
6. Once cooked, serve the hot salmon accompanied by steamed broccoli and with a squeeze of fresh lemon juice. Enjoy your meal!

34. Grilled Swordfish with Black Bean Salad

 25 minutes    1

Nutritional Values (per serving): Calories: about 290, Protein: about 20g, Fat: about 10g, Carbohydrates: about 30g, Fiber: about 4g, Sodium: about 260mg

Ingredients:
- 1 slice of swordfish
- Lemon juice
- Black pepper
- 1/2 cup black beans, drained and rinsed
- 1/4 cup corn
- 1 small tomato, diced
- 1/4 red onion, thinly sliced
- Light vinaigrette (olive oil, vinegar, mustard, salt, and pepper)

Instructions:
1. Preheat the grill to medium-high heat.
2. Season the swordfish slice with lemon juice and black pepper on both sides.
3. Grill the swordfish for about 3-4 minutes per side, or until cooked through and nicely grilled.
4. Meanwhile, prepare the black bean salad: in a large bowl, mix the drained and rinsed black beans, corn, diced tomatoes, and thinly sliced red onion.
5. Dress the salad with the light vinaigrette and toss well to combine all the ingredients.
6. Once cooked, serve the grilled swordfish hot alongside the black bean salad. Enjoy your meal!

35. Octopus Salad with Tomatoes and Olives

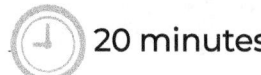 20 minutes

Nutritional Values (per serving): Calories: about 290, Protein: about 25g, Fat: about 15g, Carbohydrates: about 10g, Fiber: about 4g, Sodium: about 250mg

Ingredients:
- 150g cooked octopus
- 6-8 cherry tomatoes, halved
- 6-8 pitted black olives
- 1/4 red onion, thinly sliced
- 1 tablespoon chopped fresh parsley
- 1 tablespoon extra virgin olive oil
- 1/2 tablespoon red wine vinegar
- Salt and pepper, to taste

Instructions:
1. In a large pot, bring lightly salted water to a boil.
2. Immerse the octopus in the boiling water and cook until tender, about 15-20 minutes.
3. Drain the octopus and let it cool slightly, then cut it into pieces.
4. In a large bowl, mix the cut octopus with halved cherry tomatoes, black olives, thinly sliced red onion, and chopped fresh parsley.
5. Dress the salad with olive oil, red wine vinegar, salt, and pepper, and toss well to combine all the ingredients.
6. Let the salad rest for a few minutes to allow the flavors to meld. Serve and enjoy!
7. Bon appétit!

Vegan and Vegetarian Dishes

36. Barley and Chickpea Salad

 20 minutes  1

Nutritional Values (per serving):

Nutritions: Calories: about 290, Protein: about 10g, Fat: about 10g, Carbohydrates: about 45g, Fiber: about 6g, Sodium: about 280mg

Ingredients:
- 50g barley
- 1/2 cup cooked chickpeas
- 6-8 cherry tomatoes, halved
- 1/2 cucumber, diced
- 2 tablespoons sliced black olives, pitted
- 1 tablespoon chopped fresh parsley
- Lettuce leaves (for serving)
- 1 tablespoon olive oil
- Juice of 1/2 lemon
- 1 clove garlic, minced
- Black pepper, to taste

Instructions:
1. Cook the barley in plenty of salted water according to the package instructions. Drain it and let it cool slightly.
2. In a large bowl, combine the cooked barley, cooked chickpeas, halved cherry tomatoes, diced cucumber, sliced black olives, and chopped fresh parsley.
3. Prepare the vinaigrette by mixing together olive oil, lemon juice, minced garlic, and black pepper. Pour the vinaigrette over the salad and toss well to coat evenly.
4. Serve the barley and chickpea salad on crisp lettuce leaves and enjoy!

37. Tofu Curry with Brown Rice

 30 minutes

Nutritional Values (per serving): Calories: about 320, Fiber: about 5g, Sodium: about 290mg

Ingredients:
- 100g tofu
- 1/4 onion, chopped
- 1 teaspoon curry powder
- 1/2 bell pepper, sliced
- 1/4 cup peas
- 1/4 cup coconut milk
- 1 tomato, diced
- 1/2 cup brown rice, cooked

Instructions:
1. Cut the tofu into cubes and sauté it in a non-stick skillet with chopped onion and curry powder until golden brown.
2. Add sliced bell pepper, peas, coconut milk, and diced tomatoes to the skillet. Cook for a few minutes until the vegetables are tender and the tofu is well coated with curry.
3. Meanwhile, cook the brown rice according to the package instructions.
4. Serve the tofu curry with vegetables over cooked brown rice.

38. Roasted Vegetable Couscous

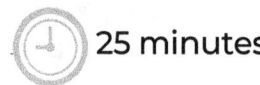 25 minutes

Nutritional Values (per serving): Calories: about 280, Protein: about 7g, Fat: about 8g, Carbohydrates: about 50g, Fiber: about 6g, Sodium: about 270mg

Ingredients:
- 50g couscous
- 1 zucchini
- 1 bell pepper
- 1/2 onion
- 1/4 eggplant
- 1 tablespoon olive oil
- 1 clove garlic, minced
- Mixed spices (e.g., oregano, thyme, chili), to taste
- Juice of 1/2 lemon
- Chopped fresh parsley

Instructions:
1. Prepare the couscous according to the package instructions and set it aside.
2. Cut the zucchini, bell pepper, onion, and eggplant into cubes or slices, according to preference.
3. Arrange the vegetables on a baking sheet and season with olive oil, minced garlic, and desired mixed spices.
4. Roast the vegetables in a preheated oven at 200°C for about 15-20 minutes or until they are tender and lightly golden.
5. In a large bowl, mix the roasted vegetables with the prepared couscous.
6. Season everything with fresh lemon juice and chopped parsley.
7. Mix well and serve the roasted vegetable couscous as a main dish or side dish.
8. Enjoy your meal!

39. Zucchini Noodles with Avocado Pesto

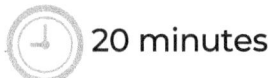 20 minutes

Nutritional Values (per serving): Calories: about 290, Protein: about 5g, Fat: about 25g, Carbohydrates: about 15g, Fiber: about 8g, Sodium: about 280mg

Ingredients:
- 1 zucchini
- 1 ripe avocado
- Fresh basil
- Juice of 1/2 lemon
- 1 clove garlic
- 1 tablespoon pine nuts
- 2 tablespoons olive oil
- 4-5 cherry tomatoes

Instructions:
1. Cut the zucchini into noodles using a spiralizer or a vegetable peeler.
2. Heat olive oil in a pan and add minced garlic. Add the zucchini noodles and sauté them until they become tender but still crisp.
3. Meanwhile, prepare the avocado pesto. In a blender, blend together ripe avocado, fresh basil, lemon juice, garlic, pine nuts, and a little olive oil until smooth and creamy.
4. Toss the zucchini noodles with the avocado pesto, mixing well to evenly coat.
5. Cut the cherry tomatoes in half and add them to the dressed zucchini noodles.
6. Serve the zucchini noodles with avocado pesto and cherry tomatoes as a main dish or side.
7. Enjoy your meal!

40. Lentil Taco

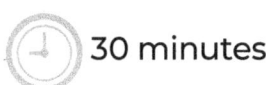 30 minutes

Nutritional Values (per serving): Calories: about 300, Protein: about 10g, Fat: about 8g, Carbohydrates: about 45g, Fiber: about 8g, Sodium: about 350mg

Ingredients:
- 50g dry lentils
- 1/4 onion, chopped
- 1 clove garlic, minced
- Mexican spices (cumin, paprika, chili powder)
- 2 whole wheat taco shells
- 1/2 avocado
- 1 small tomato
- Mixed salad greens
- 2 tablespoons tomato salsa

Instructions:
1. Cook the lentils in water or vegetable broth with chopped onion, garlic, and Mexican spices until tender and well-cooked.
2. Heat the whole wheat taco shells in the oven or in a skillet until crispy.
3. Slice the avocado and dice the tomato.
4. Prepare fresh mixed salad greens.
5. Once ready, fill the taco shells with the cooked lentils, then add avocado slices, diced tomato, and salad greens.
6. Garnish the tacos with tomato salsa and serve immediately.
7. Enjoy your meal!

41. Grilled Vegetable Wrap

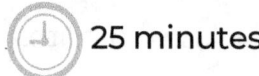 25 minutes

Nutritional Values (per serving): Calories: about 220, Protein: about 7g, Fat: about 6g, Carbohydrates: about 35g, Fiber: about 5g, Sodium: about 280mg

Ingredients:
- 1 bell pepper
- 1 zucchini
- 1 small eggplant
- 1 whole wheat tortilla
- 2 tablespoons hummus
- A handful of spinach leaves

Instructions:
1. Grill the bell pepper, zucchini, and eggplant until tender and lightly charred. Once done, slice them into strips.
2. Spread a layer of hummus over the whole wheat tortilla.
3. Arrange the spinach leaves on the tortilla with hummus.
4. Evenly distribute the grilled vegetable strips on top of the spinach leaves.
5. Roll the tortilla with the vegetables inside to form a wrap.
6. Cut the wrap in half and serve immediately.
7. Enjoy your meal!

42. Corn Tortillas with Beans and Salsa

 20 minutes

Nutritional Values (per serving): Calories: about 260, Protein: about 8g, Fat: about 2g, Carbohydrates: about 50g, Fiber: about 5g, Sodium: about 290mg

Ingredients:
- 2 corn tortillas
- 1/2 cup cooked black beans
- 1/4 cup sweet corn
- 1/4 bell pepper, diced
- 1 small tomato, diced
- 2 tablespoons fresh tomato salsa
- Fresh cilantro, chopped (for garnish)

Instructions:
1. Heat the corn tortillas in a skillet or microwave until they are soft and flexible.
2. Fill each tortilla with cooked black beans, sweet corn, diced bell pepper, and diced tomato.
3. Roll up the filled tortillas to form wraps.
4. Serve the tortillas with fresh tomato salsa.
5. Garnish with chopped fresh cilantro and serve.
6. Enjoy your meal!

SOUPS AND BROTHS

43. Vegetable Soup

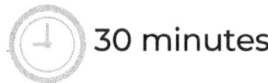 30 minutes

Nutritional Values (per serving): Calories: about 120, Carbohydrates: about 20g, Protein: about 7g, Fat: about 4g, Fiber: about 5g, Sodium: about 200mg

Ingredients:
- 1/2 onion, diced
- 1 clove garlic, minced
- 1 tablespoon olive oil
- 1 carrot, diced
- 1 stalk celery, diced
- 1/2 zucchini, diced
- 2 cups vegetable broth

Instructions:
1. In a pot, heat olive oil over medium heat.
2. Add diced onion and minced garlic, sauté for a few minutes until golden and fragrant.
3. Add diced carrots, celery, and zucchini to the pot, and mix well with the onion and garlic.
4. Pour vegetable broth over the vegetables in the pot, ensuring they are covered.
5. Bring the broth to a boil, then reduce the heat and let the soup simmer for about 20-25 minutes or until the vegetables are tender.
6. Once the vegetables are cooked, taste the soup and adjust salt and pepper according to your personal preference.
7. Serve the hot vegetable soup and enjoy it on its own or with some breadsticks.
8. Enjoy your meal!

44. Lentil Soup

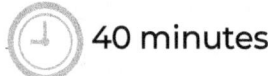 40 minutes

Nutritional Values (per serving): Calories: about 150, Carbohydrates: about 25g, Protein: about 7g, Fat: about 7g, Fiber: about 8g, Sodium: about 220mg

Ingredients:
- 1/2 onion, diced
- 1 stalk celery, diced
- 1 tablespoon olive oil
- 1/2 cup dry lentils
- 2 cups vegetable broth

Instructions:
1. In a pot, heat olive oil over medium heat.
2. Add diced onion and diced celery, sauté for a few minutes until golden and soft.
3. Add dry lentils to the pot and mix well with the onion and celery.
4. Pour vegetable broth over the lentils, making sure they are completely immersed.
5. Bring the broth to a boil, then reduce the heat and let the soup simmer for about 30-35 minutes or until the lentils are soft.
6. Once the lentils are cooked, taste the soup and adjust salt and pepper according to your personal preference.
7. Serve the hot lentil soup and enjoy it on its own or with some breadsticks.
8. Enjoy your meal!

45. Minestrone with Barley

 35 minutes

Nutritions: Calories: Approximately 140 kcal, Protein: Approximately 5-7g, Fat: Approximately 3-5g, Carbohydrates: Approximately 25-30g, Fiber: Approximately 6-8g, Sodium: Approximately 210mg

Ingredients:
- 1 medium onion, diced
- 2 medium carrots, diced
- 2 tablespoons olive oil
- 400g diced tomatoes (canned or fresh)
- 400g drained cannellini beans (canned)
- 100g barley
- 1 liter vegetable broth
- Salt and pepper to taste
- Chopped fresh parsley (optional, for garnish)

Instructions:
1. Heat olive oil in a large pot over medium heat. Add diced onion and diced carrots, and sauté until softened, stirring occasionally for about 5-7 minutes.
2. Add diced tomatoes, drained cannellini beans, and barley to the pot. Mix well.
3. Pour vegetable broth into the pot and bring it to a boil.
4. Reduce the heat and let the minestrone simmer over medium-low heat for about 20-25 minutes, or until the vegetables and barley are tender. Stir occasionally during cooking.
5. Taste the minestrone and adjust salt and pepper to your liking.
6. Once the minestrone is ready, turn off the heat and let it rest for a few minutes before serving.
7. Ladle the minestrone into bowls and garnish with chopped fresh parsley if desired.
8. Enjoy your hot minestrone, with some crusty bread or breadsticks if you prefer.

46. Pumpkin and Carrot Soup

Approximate Nutritional Values (per serving): Calories: about 130, Protein: 2g, Fat: 1g, Carbohydrates: 28g, Fiber: 6g, Sodium: 200mg

Ingredients:
- 500g pumpkin, peeled and diced
- 2 medium carrots, peeled and sliced
- 1 liter vegetable broth
- Salt and pepper, to taste
- Fresh chopped parsley (optional, for garnish)

Instructions:
1. Prepare the vegetables: peel and dice the pumpkin and slice the carrots.
2. Steam the pumpkin and carrots until they are tender. This may take about 20-25 minutes, depending on the size of the pieces.
3. Once cooked, transfer the pumpkin and carrots to a blender or immersion blender.
4. Add about half of the vegetable broth to the blender along with the cooked vegetables.
5. Blend the vegetables and broth until smooth and creamy. If the soup is too thick, gradually add the remaining broth until reaching the desired consistency.
6. Pour the blended soup into a pot and heat it over medium-low heat. Season with salt and pepper to taste.
7. Once heated, distribute the soup into bowls.
8. Garnish with fresh chopped parsley, if desired, before serving.
9. Serve the soup hot with breadsticks or crusty bread, if preferred.

47. Pea and Mint Soup

Approximate Nutritional Values (per serving): Calories: about 120, Protein: 4g, Fat: 5g, Carbohydrates: 14g, Fiber: 5g, Sodium: 190mg

Ingredients:
- 1 medium onion, finely chopped
- 2 celery stalks, diced
- 2 cups fresh or frozen peas
- 4 cups vegetable broth
- 2 tablespoons olive oil
- 1/4 cup fresh mint leaves, finely chopped
- Salt and freshly ground black pepper, to taste

Instructions:
1. Begin by preparing the Ingredients:
2. finely chop the onion, dice the celery, and finely chop the mint leaves.
3. In a large pot, heat the olive oil over medium heat. Add the chopped onion and diced celery and sauté for about 5-7 minutes, until softened and translucent.
4. Add the fresh or frozen peas to the pot and stir well with the onions and celery. Continue to cook for another 2-3 minutes.
5. Pour the vegetable broth into the pot with the peas. Bring it to a boil, then reduce the heat and let it simmer gently for about 15-20 minutes, or until the peas are tender.
6. Once the peas are tender, remove the pot from the heat. Add the chopped mint leaves and stir well.
7. Using an immersion blender or a traditional blender, blend the soup until smooth and creamy.
8. Taste and adjust seasoning with salt and pepper, if necessary, according to your personal preference.
9. Once you've achieved the desired consistency, return the soup to the heat and warm it over medium-low heat for a few minutes, stirring occasionally.
10. When the soup is hot, serve it in individual bowls and garnish with a few fresh mint leaves.

48. Spinach and Potato Soup

Approximate Nutritional Values (per serving): Calories: about 140, Protein: 4g, Fat: 1g, Carbohydrates: 30g, Fiber: 6g, Sodium: 200mg

Ingredients:
- 2 medium potatoes, peeled and cubed
- 200g fresh spinach
- 4 cups vegetable broth
- Salt and freshly ground black pepper, to taste

Instructions:
1. Start by preparing the Ingredients:
2. peel and cube the potatoes, then thoroughly wash and drain the fresh spinach.
3. Place the potato cubes in a steaming basket and steam them until tender, about 15-20 minutes. You can also boil the diced potatoes in a pot of boiling water, but steaming preserves nutrients better.
4. While the potatoes are cooking, prepare the vegetable broth if you haven't already.
5. Once the potatoes are tender, transfer them to a blender along with the fresh spinach and 2 cups of vegetable broth. Blend until smooth.
6. Pour the potato and spinach puree into a pot, add the remaining 2 cups of vegetable broth, and mix well. Bring the soup to medium-low heat and let it simmer for about 5-10 minutes, stirring occasionally.
7. Taste the soup and adjust the seasoning with salt and pepper, if necessary, according to your personal preference.
8. Once the soup is hot and the flavors have melded, serve it in individual bowls.
9. You can garnish the soup with a sprinkle of freshly ground black pepper and some fresh parsley leaves, if desired.

49. Caramelized Onion Soup

Approximate Nutritional Values (per serving): Calories: about 160, Protein: 2g, Fat: 7g, Carbohydrates: 22g, Fiber: 4g, Sodium: 220mg

Ingredients:
- 4 medium onions, sliced
- 2 tablespoons olive oil
- 4 cups vegetable broth
- 1 tablespoon fresh thyme leaves
- Salt and freshly ground black pepper, to taste

Instructions:
1. Begin by preparing the Ingredients:
2. peel and thinly slice the onions, then wash and dry the fresh thyme leaves.
3. In a large pot, heat the olive oil over medium heat. Add the sliced onions and gently caramelize them, stirring occasionally, until they become soft and golden, about 20-30 minutes. Make sure not to let them burn; adjust the heat if necessary.
4. Once the onions are caramelized, add the vegetable broth and fresh thyme leaves. Mix well to incorporate the ingredients.
5. Bring the soup to a boil, then reduce the heat and let it simmer gently for about 15-20 minutes, or until the onions have become tender and the flavors have melded.
6. Taste the soup and adjust the seasoning with salt and pepper according to your personal preference.
7. Once the soup is ready, turn off the heat and let it cool slightly before serving.
8. Ladle the caramelized onion soup into individual bowls and garnish with a sprinkle of freshly ground black pepper, if desired.
9. Serve the soup hot and accompany it with whole grain bread toast, if desired.

50. Lentil and Tomato Soup

Approximate Nutritional Values (per serving): Calories: about 150, Protein: 8g, Fat: 1g, Carbohydrates: 30g, Fiber: 6g, Sodium: 220mg

Ingredients:
- 1 cup red lentils
- 2 cups diced tomatoes
- 1 onion, chopped
- 2 cloves garlic, minced
- 4 cups vegetable broth
- Lemon juice, for serving
- Salt and freshly ground black pepper, to taste
- Olive oil, for sautéing vegetables (optional)

Instructions:
1. First, prepare the Ingredients: rinse the lentils thoroughly under running water and drain. Finely chop the onion and garlic, and dice the tomatoes if you haven't already.
2. In a large pot, heat a little olive oil (optional) over medium heat. Add the chopped onion and garlic and sauté for a few minutes until they become translucent and fragrant.
3. Add the diced tomatoes to the pot and mix well with the onions and garlic. Let them cook for about 5-7 minutes until the tomatoes slightly soften.
4. Add the red lentils to the pot and mix well with the sautéed vegetables. Toast the lentils for a couple of minutes, then pour the vegetable broth into the pot.
5. Bring the soup to a boil, then reduce the heat and let it simmer gently for about 25-30 minutes, or until the lentils are soft and the soup has reached the desired consistency. During cooking, stir occasionally and add more broth if necessary.
6. Taste the soup and adjust the seasoning with salt and pepper according to your personal preference.
7. Once the soup is ready, turn off the heat and let it cool slightly before serving.
8. Ladle the hot lentil soup into individual bowls and add a squeeze of fresh lemon juice to each portion for a touch of freshness.

51. Pumpkin and Ginger Soup

Approximate Nutritional Values (per serving): Calories: about 140, Protein: 2g, Fat: 6g, Carbohydrates: 20g, Fiber: 4g, Sodium: 190mg

Ingredients:
- 250g pumpkin, peeled and diced
- 1/2 onion, chopped
- 1 tablespoon grated fresh ginger
- 2 cups vegetable broth
- 1/4 cup coconut milk (optional)
- Salt and freshly ground black pepper, to taste
- Olive oil, for sautéing vegetables (optional)

Instructions:
1. First, prepare the Ingredients: peel the pumpkin and cut it into cubes. Finely chop the onion and grate the fresh ginger.
2. In a large pot, heat a little olive oil (optional) over medium heat. Add the chopped onion and grated ginger and sauté for a few minutes until they become fragrant.
3. Add the pumpkin cubes to the pot and mix well with the onions and ginger. Let them cook for about 5-7 minutes until the pumpkin begins to soften slightly.
4. Pour the vegetable broth into the pot and bring it to a boil. Reduce the heat and let it simmer over medium-low heat for about 20-25 minutes, or until the pumpkin is completely tender.
5. Once the pumpkin is soft, use an immersion blender to blend the soup directly in the pot until it reaches a creamy and smooth consistency.
6. If you desire a creamier and richer soup, add the coconut milk to the soup and mix well.
7. Taste the soup and adjust the seasoning with salt and pepper according to your personal preference.
8. Once the soup is ready, turn off the heat and let it cool slightly before serving. Enjoy your meal!

52. Cauliflower and Curry Soup

Nutritional Values (per approximate serving): Calories: about 150, Protein: 4g, Fat: 2g, Carbohydrates: 30g, Fiber: 5g, Sodium: 210mg

Ingredients:
- 1 medium cauliflower, divided into florets
- 1 onion, chopped
- 2 teaspoons curry powder
- 4 cups vegetable broth
- Salt and freshly ground black pepper, to taste
- Fresh coriander leaves, for garnish

Instructions:
1. First, prepare the Ingredients:
2. divide the cauliflower into florets, finely chop the onion, and gather the curry powder.
3. In a large pot, heat a little olive oil (optional) over medium heat. Add the chopped onion and sauté for a few minutes until it becomes translucent and soft.
4. Add the cauliflower florets to the pot along with the onion and mix well to evenly distribute the onion and curry.
5. Continue to cook for about 5 minutes, stirring occasionally, until the cauliflower begins to soften slightly and the curry releases its aroma.
6. Pour the vegetable broth into the pot and bring to a boil. Reduce the heat and let it simmer over medium-low heat for about 20-25 minutes, or until the cauliflower is completely tender.
7. Once the cauliflower is tender, use an immersion blender to blend the soup directly in the pot until it reaches a smooth and creamy consistency.
8. Taste the soup and adjust the seasoning with salt and pepper according to your personal preference.
9. Once the soup is ready, turn off the heat and serve it hot.
10. Garnish with fresh coriander leaves before serving and enjoy this delicious cauliflower and curry soup!

SALADS AND SIDES

SALADS

53. Spinach and Strawberry Salad

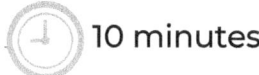 10 minutes

Nutritional Values: Calories: about 180 per serving, Fiber: 5g, Sodium: 250mg, Badge: Vegan

Operational Instructions:
1. Toss together fresh spinach, sliced strawberries, and slivered almonds.
2. Dress with a light vinaigrette made with balsamic vinegar, olive oil, and a teaspoon of honey.

54. Quinoa Salad with Roasted Vegetables

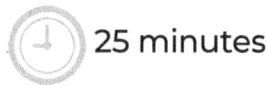 25 minutes

Nutritional Values: Calories: about 230 per serving, Fiber: 6g, Sodium: 280mg, Badge: Vegan

Operational Instructions:
1. Cook quinoa and let it cool.
2. Add diced roasted zucchini and bell peppers, halved cherry tomatoes, and fresh parsley.
3. Dress with olive oil, lemon juice, minced garlic, and black pepper.

55. Black Bean and Corn Salad

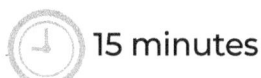 15 minutes

Nutritional Values: Calories: about 220 per serving, Fiber: 7g, Sodium: 290mg, Badge: Vegan

Operational Instructions:
1. Mix cooked black beans, sweet corn, diced bell peppers, and thinly sliced red onion.
2. Dress with fresh lime juice, chopped cilantro, olive oil, and a pinch of chili powder.

56. Chickpea and Tomato Salad

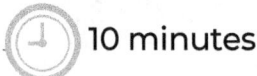 10 minutes

Nutritional Values: Calories: about 190 per serving, Fiber: 5g, Sodium: 270mg, Badge: Vegan

Operational Instructions:
1. Combine cooked chickpeas, diced tomatoes, cubed cucumbers, and fresh parsley.
2. Dress with apple cider vinegar, olive oil, minced garlic, and a sprinkle of oregano.

57. Cucumber and Melon Salad

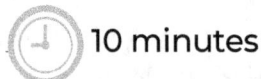 10 minutes

Nutritional Values: Calories: about 180 per serving, Fiber: 3g, Sodium: 250mg, Badge: Vegan

Operational Instructions:
1. Mix thinly sliced cucumbers, diced melon, and fresh mint leaves.
2. Dress with fresh lime juice and a light sprinkle of sea salt.

58. Beet and Cucumber Salad

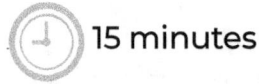 15 minutes

Nutritional Values: Calories: about 190 per serving, Fiber: 4g, Sodium: 260mg, Badge: Vegan

Operational Instructions:
1. Boil the beets, then peel and slice them thinly.
2. Toss with thinly sliced cucumbers, fresh mint leaves, and chopped walnuts.
3. Dress with red wine vinegar, olive oil, black pepper, and a splash of lemon juice.

59. Farro Salad with Cherry Tomatoes and Olives

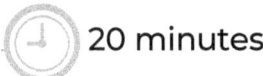 20 minutes

Nutritional Values: Calories: about 220 per serving, Fiber: 5g, Sodium: 270mg, Badge: Vegetarian

Operational Instructions:
1. Cook the farro and let it cool.
2. Add halved cherry tomatoes, sliced black olives, and thinly sliced red onion.
3. Dress with balsamic vinegar, olive oil, minced garlic, and fresh basil.

60. Roasted Tomato and Cucumber Salad

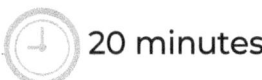 20 minutes

Nutritional Values: Calories: about 200 per serving, Fiber: 4g, Sodium: 270mg, Badge: Vegan

Operational Instructions:
1. Cut the tomatoes in half and roast them in the oven until soft.
2. Mix with thinly sliced cucumbers, thinly sliced red onion, and fresh basil.
3. Dress with red wine vinegar, olive oil, minced garlic, and a sprinkle of oregano.

61. Couscous and Vegetable Salad

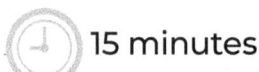 15 minutes

Nutritional Values: Calories: about 210 per serving, Fiber: 5g, Sodium: 280mg, Badge: Vegan

Operational Instructions:
1. Prepare the couscous according to the package instructions and let it cool.
2. Add diced bell peppers, cucumbers, and cherry tomatoes.
3. Dress with fresh lemon juice, chopped cilantro, olive oil, and black pepper.

62. Green Bean and Almond Salad

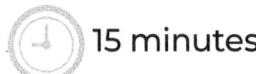 15 minutes

Nutritional Values: Calories: about 220 per serving, Fiber: 6g, Sodium: 270mg, Badge: Vegan

Operational Instructions:
1. Blanch the green beans until tender but crisp.
2. Mix with sliced almonds, diced cherry tomatoes, and chopped fresh parsley.
3. Dress with apple cider vinegar, olive oil, minced garlic, and a sprinkle of black pepper.

Side Dishes

63. Chickpea and Tomato Salad

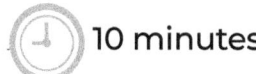 10 minutes

Nutritional Values: Calories: about 150 per serving, Fiber: 6g, Sodium: 180mg, Badge: Vegan

Operational Instructions:
1. Drain and rinse canned chickpeas, then mix them with halved cherry tomatoes.
2. Dress with olive oil, balsamic vinegar, chopped fresh parsley, salt, and pepper.

64. Sautéed Spinach with Garlic and Lemon

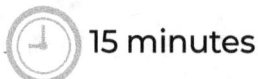 15 minutes

Nutritional Values: Calories: about 70 per serving, Fiber: 4g, Sodium: 180mg, Badge: Vegan

Operational Instructions:
1. Heat a non-stick skillet and sauté spinach with minced garlic and lemon juice until wilted.

65. Roasted Sweet Potatoes

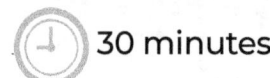 30 minutes

Nutritional Values: Calories: about 120 per serving, Fiber: 4g, Sodium: 220mg, Badge: Vegan

Operational Instructions:
1. Dice sweet potatoes and toss with olive oil, paprika, salt, and pepper.
2. Roast in the oven at 200°C until golden brown.

66. Steamed Broccoli with Almonds

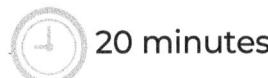 15 minutes

Nutritional Values: Calories: about 90 per serving, Fiber: 5g, Sodium: 190mg, Badge: Vegan

Operational Instructions:
1. Steam broccoli until tender, then sprinkle with chopped toasted almonds and a drizzle of olive oil.

67. Quinoa and Vegetable Salad

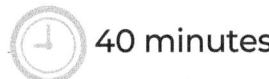 20 minutes

Nutritional Values: Calories: about 180 per serving, Fiber: 6g, Sodium: 200mg, Badge: Vegan

Operational Instructions:
1. Cook the quinoa and let it cool, then mix it with grilled vegetables such as bell peppers, zucchini, and red onions.
2. Dress with olive oil, lemon juice, salt, and pepper.

68. Cauliflower Gratin

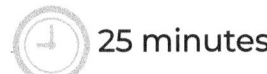 40 minutes

Nutritional Values: Calories: about 130 per serving, Fiber: 5g, Sodium: 210mg, Badge: Vegan

Operational Instructions:
1. Steam the cauliflower until tender, then transfer it to a baking dish.
2. Cover with a light white sauce and bake in the oven until golden brown.

69. Beet and Chickpea Salad

25 minutes

Nutritional Values: Calories: about 160 per serving, Fiber: 7g, Sodium: 220mg, Badge: Vegan

Operational Instructions:
1. Cook the beets, then peel and dice them.
2. Mix with cooked chickpeas, chopped fresh parsley, and dress with olive oil, red wine vinegar, salt, and pepper.

70. Cucumber and Avocado Salad

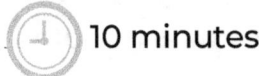 10 minutes

Nutritional Values: Calories: about 140 per serving, Fiber: 5g, Sodium: 170mg, Badge: Vegan

Operational Instructions:
1. Dice cucumbers and avocados, then mix them together.
2. Dress with lime juice, chopped fresh cilantro, salt, and pepper.

71. Grilled Zucchini with Basil Pesto

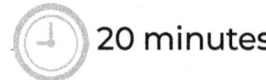 20 minutes

Nutritional Values: Calories: about 110 per serving, Fiber: 4g, Sodium: 200mg, Badge: Vegan

Operational Instructions:
1. Slice the zucchini into thin slices and grill them until tender.
2. Dress with homemade basil pesto.

72. Green Beans with Almonds and Lemon

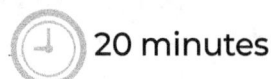 20 minutes

Nutritional Values: Calories: about 100 per serving, Fiber: 4g, Sodium: 180mg, Badge: Vegan

Operational Instructions:
1. Steam the green beans until al dente.
2. Sauté the beans in a pan with chopped almonds and lemon juice.

73. Arugula and Strawberry Salad

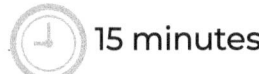 15 minutes

Nutritional Values: Calories: about 90 per serving, Fiber: 3g, Sodium: 160mg, Badge: Vegan

Operational Instructions:
1. Mix fresh arugula with sliced strawberries.
2. Dress with reduced balsamic vinegar and freshly ground black pepper.

74. Grilled Eggplant with Parsley Pesto

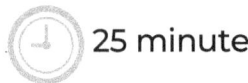 25 minutes

Nutritional Values: Calories: about 110 per serving, Fiber: 4g, Sodium: 180mg, Badge: Vegan

Operational Instructions:
1. Slice the eggplant into rounds and grill them until soft.
2. Dress with a fresh pesto made with parsley, garlic, olive oil, and walnuts.

75. Artichokes Gratin with Breadcrumbs and Lemon

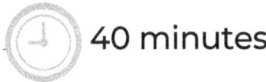 40 minutes

Nutritional Values: Calories: about 130 per serving, Fiber: 5g, Sodium: 200mg, Badge: Vegan

Operational Instructions:
1. Steam the artichoke hearts until tender.
2. Sprinkle with breadcrumbs seasoned with grated lemon zest and chopped parsley, then gratin in the oven until golden brown.

Dear Reader,

We hope that our Cookbook is taking you on an exciting culinary journey, enriching your days with delicious and healthy dishes. We would cordially invite you to share your experience with us and other readers by leaving a review on Amazon.

Your opinions are extremely important to us. By sharing your impressions of the book, you help us improve and offer content that is increasingly tailored to your needs and tastes.

Fast fuel fast food

76. Grilled Chicken Sandwich and Baked Potato Chips

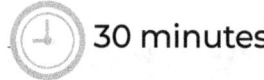 30 minutes

Nutritional Values (per serving): Calories: about 400, Protein: about 25g, Fat: about 15g, Carbohydrates: about 40g, Fiber: about 5g, Sodium: about 450mg

Ingredients:
- 1 chicken breast
- 1 sandwich bun
- Lettuce leaves
- Sliced tomato
- Pickled cucumbers
- Olive oil
- Minced garlic
- Lemon juice
- Black pepper
- Salt
- Potatoes
- Chopped parsley (optional, for garnish)

Instructions:
1. Marinate the chicken breast with some olive oil, minced garlic, lemon juice, and black pepper, ensuring it's well coated. Let it marinate for at least 15-20 minutes.
2. Grill the marinated chicken breast over medium-high heat until golden brown and fully cooked. Make sure the chicken reaches an adequate internal temperature for food safety.
3. Meanwhile, slice the sandwich bun in half and lightly toast it on a skillet or in the oven.
4. Prepare the baked potato chips: peel and thinly slice the potatoes, then season them with a drizzle of olive oil, salt, and pepper. Arrange them on a baking sheet and bake at 200°C for about 20-25 minutes, flipping halfway through, until crispy and golden brown.
5. Once cooked, assemble the sandwich: layer lettuce leaves, tomato slices, and pickled cucumbers on the toasted bun.
6. Add the grilled chicken breast to the sandwich and serve accompanied by the baked potato chips.
7. If desired, garnish the sandwich with some chopped parsley before serving.

77. Vegetarian Sandwich with Hummus and Baked Potato Chips

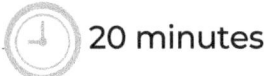 20 minutes

Nutritional Values (per serving): Calories: about 350, Protein: about 8g, Fat: about 15g, Carbohydrates: about 45g, Fiber: about 6g, Sodium: about 400mg

Ingredients:
- 1 whole grain sandwich bun
- Hummus
- 1 cucumber
- 1 bell pepper
- 1 carrot
- Fresh spinach leaves
- 1 ripe avocado
- Baked potato chips
- Paprika
- Salt

Instructions:
1. Spread some hummus on both halves of the sandwich bun.
2. Thinly slice the cucumber, bell pepper, and carrot.
3. Arrange the cucumber, bell pepper, and carrot slices on the bun over the hummus layer.
4. Add some fresh spinach leaves over the vegetables.
5. Slice the ripe avocado and distribute the slices over the spinach leaves.
6. Season the baked potato chips with paprika and salt.
7. Serve the vegan sandwich with hummus and vegetables alongside the seasoned baked potato chips.

78. Turkey Burger Sandwich with Roasted Potato Wedges

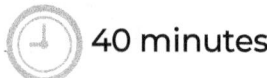 40 minutes

Nutritional Values (per serving): Calories: about 420, Protein: about 25g, Fat: about 20g, Carbohydrates: about 35g, Fiber: about 4g, Sodium: about 480mg

Ingredients:

- 1 sandwich bun
- 150g ground turkey meat
- 1/4 finely chopped onion
- 1 clove garlic, minced
- 1 tablespoon fresh parsley, chopped
- Salt and pepper to taste
- Sliced cheese (of choice)
- Lettuce
- Tomato
- Potatoes
- Rosemary
- Garlic powder
- Olive oil

Instructions:

1. In a bowl, mix ground turkey meat with finely chopped onion, minced garlic, fresh parsley, salt, and pepper. Form patties with the mixture.
2. Cook the turkey burgers in a pan with a drizzle of olive oil until golden brown and cooked through, about 5-6 minutes per side over medium heat.
3. Meanwhile, slice the sandwich bun in half and lightly toast it.
4. Once ready, place the turkey burgers on the buns and add cheese slices, lettuce, and tomato slices.
5. For the roasted potato wedges, cut the potatoes into wedges and place them on a baking tray. Season with olive oil, chopped fresh rosemary, and garlic powder. Bake in a preheated oven at 200°C for about 25-30 minutes, or until the potatoes are golden and crispy.
6. Serve the turkey burger sandwich with freshly cooked roasted potato wedges.

79. BLT Sandwich with Paprika Potato Chips

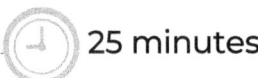 25 minutes

Nutritional Values (per serving): Calories: about 380, Protein: about 10g, Fat: about 20g, Carbohydrates: about 40g, Fiber: about 4g, Sodium: about 420mg

Ingredients:
- 1 sandwich bun
- 2 bacon slices
- Lettuce
- Tomato
- Potatoes
- Olive oil
- Paprika
- Salt and pepper

Instructions:
1. In a non-stick skillet, cook the bacon slices until crispy. Once ready, set them aside on paper towels to remove excess fat.
2. Slice the sandwich bun in half and lightly toast it, if preferred.
3. Add the crispy bacon slices on the base of the bun.
4. Add lettuce leaves and tomato slices over the bacon.
5. For the paprika potato chips, preheat the oven to 200°C. Cut the potatoes into wedges and place them on a baking tray lined with parchment paper. Season the potatoes with olive oil, paprika, salt, and pepper, tossing well to evenly distribute the spices.
6. Bake the potato chips in the preheated oven for about 20-25 minutes, flipping halfway through, until golden and crispy.
7. Serve the BLT sandwich with freshly cooked paprika potato chips.

80. Philly Cheese Steak Sandwich with Thyme Potato Wedges

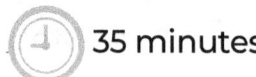 35 minutes

Nutritional Values (per serving): Calories: about 450, Protein: about 20g, Fat: about 20g, Carbohydrates: about 45g, Fiber: about 5g, Sodium: about 470mg

Ingredients:
- 100g beef slices (thinly sliced)
- 1/4 onion (sliced)
- 1/4 bell pepper (sliced)
- 1 sandwich bun
- Sliced cheese (Provolone or American cheese)
- 1 potato
- Olive oil
- Fresh thyme
- Salt and pepper

Instructions:
1. In a non-stick skillet, cook the beef slices together with sliced onion and bell pepper until the beef is cooked and the vegetables are tender.
2. Slice the sandwich bun in half and lightly toast it.
3. Fill the bun with the cooked beef, evenly distributing cheese slices over the beef.
4. Cover the skillet with a lid to melt the cheese.
5. Meanwhile, prepare the thyme potato wedges: preheat the oven to 200°C. Cut the potato into thin slices and place them on a baking tray lined with parchment paper. Season the potatoes with olive oil, fresh thyme leaves, salt, and pepper, tossing well to evenly coat with the spices.
6. Bake the potato wedges in the preheated oven for about 20-25 minutes or until golden and crispy.
7. Serve the Philly Cheese Steak Sandwich with freshly cooked thyme potato wedges.

PIZZAS

Dough

81. Whole Wheat Pizza Dough

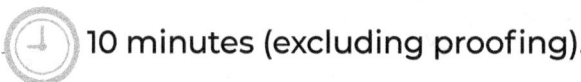 10 minutes (excluding proofing).

Nutritional Values (per serving of dough): Calories: 150 kcal, Fiber: 3g, Sodium: 230mg., Badge: Vegetarian.

Ingredients:
- whole wheat flour, brewer's yeast, warm water, olive oil, salt.

Operating Instructions:
1. Mix whole wheat flour with brewer's yeast and salt. Add olive oil and warm water, then knead until smooth. Let it proof for at least an hour.

82. Chickpea Flour Pizza Dough

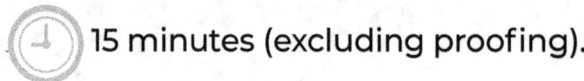 15 minutes (excluding proofing).

Nutritional Values (per serving of dough): Calories: 160 kcal, Fiber: 4g, Sodium: 240mg., Badge: Vegetarian.

Ingredients:
- chickpea flour, durum wheat flour, brewer's yeast, warm water, salt.

Operating Instructions:
1. Mix flours with brewer's yeast and salt. Add warm water and knead until elastic. Let it proof for at least an hour.

83. Oat Flour Pizza Dough

🕐 10 minutes (excluding proofing).

Nutritional Values (per serving of dough): Calories: 140 kcal, Fiber: 2g, Sodium: 220mg, Badge: Vegetarian.

Ingredients:
- oat flour, brewer's yeast, warm water, extra virgin olive oil, salt.

Operating Instructions:
1. Mix oat flour with brewer's yeast and salt. Add extra virgin olive oil and warm water, then knead until soft. Let it proof for at least an hour.

84. Corn Flour Pizza Dough

🕐 15 minutes (excluding proofing).

Nutritional Values (per serving of dough): Calories: 170 kcal, Fiber: 3.5g, Sodium: 250mg, Badge: Vegetarian.

Ingredients:
- corn flour, durum wheat flour, brewer's yeast, warm water, salt.

Operating Instructions:
1. Mix flours with brewer's yeast and salt. Add warm water and knead until elastic. Let it proof for at least an hour.

85. Coconut Flour Pizza Dough

🕐 15 minutes (excluding proofing).

Nutritional Values (per serving of dough): Calories: 180 kcal, Fiber: 5g, Sodium: 260mg, Badge: Vegetarian.

Ingredients:
- coconut flour, durum wheat flour, brewer's yeast, warm water, extra virgin olive oil, salt.

Operating Instructions:
1. Mix flours with brewer's yeast and salt. Add extra virgin olive oil and warm water, then knead until smooth. Let it proof for at least an hour.

86. Buckwheat Flour Pizza Dough

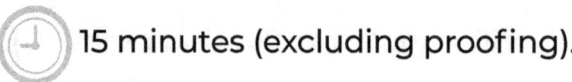 15 minutes (excluding proofing).

Nutritional Values (per serving of dough): Calories: 190 kcal, Fiber: 4g, Sodium: 280mg, Badge: Vegetarian.

Ingredients:
- 1 cup buckwheat flour, 1 cup durum wheat flour, 1 packet brewer's yeast, 1 cup warm water, 2 tablespoons extra virgin olive oil, 1 teaspoon salt.

Operating Instructions:
1. In a large bowl, mix flours, brewer's yeast, and salt. Add warm water and extra virgin olive oil, then knead until soft and homogeneous. Cover with a damp cloth and let it proof for at least an hour in a warm place. Once proofed, the dough is ready to be rolled out and topped to make the pizza.

87. Light Margherita Pizza

 20 minutes (including baking time)

Nutritional Values (per serving): Calories: 250 kcal, Protein: 12g, Fat: 7g, Carbohydrates: 35g, Fiber: 3g, Sodium: 300mg, **Badge:** Vegetarian

Ingredients (for one person):
- Whole wheat pizza base
- 2 tablespoons of unsweetened tomato sauce
- 50g of light mozzarella, thinly sliced
- Fresh basil leaves, to taste

Instructions:
1. Preheat the oven to 200°C (about 400°F).
2. Roll out the whole wheat pizza base on a lightly greased baking sheet or lined with parchment paper.
3. Spread the tomato sauce evenly over the pizza base, leaving a border around the edges.
4. Arrange the slices of light mozzarella on top of the tomato sauce.
5. Add the fresh basil leaves evenly over the mozzarella.
6. Place the pizza in the preheated oven and bake for about 12-15 minutes, or until the crust is golden brown and the cheese is melted and slightly golden.
7. Once cooked, remove the pizza from the oven and let it cool slightly before slicing and serving.
8. Enjoy your delicious Light Margherita Pizza with a crispy whole wheat crust and a light, flavorful topping! Bon Appétit!

88. Vegetarian Pizza with Grilled Vegetables

 25 minutes (including cooking time)

Nutritional Information (per serving): Calories: 280 kcal, Protein: 8g, Fat: 4g, Carbohydrates: 45g, Fiber: 7g, Sodium: 320mg

Ingredients (for one serving):
- 1 whole wheat pizza base
- 3 tablespoons unsweetened tomato sauce
- 1/4 cup grilled eggplant slices
- 1/4 cup roasted bell peppers
- 1/4 cup sliced zucchini
- 1/4 cup caramelized onions

Instructions:
1. Preheat the oven to 200°C (approximately 400°F).
2. Spread the unsweetened tomato sauce evenly over the whole wheat pizza base.
3. Arrange the grilled eggplant slices, roasted bell peppers, sliced zucchini, and caramelized onions on top of the tomato sauce.
4. Place the pizza in the preheated oven and bake for about 15-18 minutes or until the crust is golden brown and the vegetables are tender.
5. Once baked, remove the pizza from the oven and let it cool for a few minutes.
6. Slice the pizza into portions and serve hot.
7. Enjoy your delicious Vegetarian Pizza with Grilled Vegetables!

89. Pizza with Chicken and Spinach

 25 minutes (including baking time)

Nutritional Information (per serving): Calories: 280 kcal, Protein: 7g, Fat: 4g, Carbohydrates: 50g, Fiber: 5g, Sodium: 320mg

Ingredients (for one serving):
- 1 whole wheat pizza base
- 3 tablespoons unsweetened tomato sauce
- 1/4 cup grilled eggplant slices
- 1/4 cup roasted bell peppers
- 1/4 cup sliced zucchini
- 2 tablespoons caramelized onions

Instructions:
1. Preheat the oven to 200°C (approximately 400°F).
2. Spread the unsweetened tomato sauce evenly over the whole wheat pizza base.
3. Arrange the grilled eggplant slices, roasted bell peppers, sliced zucchini, and caramelized onions on top of the tomato sauce.
4. Place the pizza in the preheated oven and bake for about 15-18 minutes or until the crust is golden brown and the toppings are cooked.
5. Once baked, remove the pizza from the oven and let it cool for a few minutes.
6. Slice the pizza into portions and serve hot.
7. Enjoy your delicious Vegetarian Pizza with Grilled Vegetables!

90. Pizza with Tuna and Capers

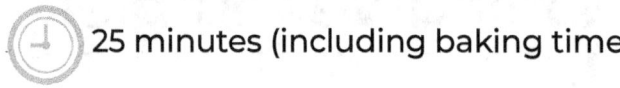 25 minutes (including baking time)

Nutritional Information (per serving): Calories: 270 kcal, Protein: 20g, Fat: 9g, Carbohydrates: 25g, Fiber: 3.5g, Sodium: 320mg

Ingredients (for one serving):
- 1 whole wheat pizza base
- 3 tablespoons unsweetened tomato sauce
- 1/2 cup drained canned tuna
- 2 tablespoons capers
- 1 medium-sized tomato, thinly sliced

Instructions:
1. Preheat the oven to 200°C (approximately 400°F).
2. Spread the unsweetened tomato sauce evenly over the whole wheat pizza base.
3. Distribute the drained canned tuna and capers evenly on top of the tomato sauce.
4. Place the thinly sliced tomatoes on the pizza.
5. Place the pizza in the preheated oven and bake for about 12-15 minutes or until the crust is golden brown and the toppings are cooked.
6. Once baked, remove the pizza from the oven and let it cool for a few minutes.
7. Slice the pizza into portions and serve hot.
8. Enjoy your delicious Pizza with Tuna and Capers!

91. Pizza with Mushrooms and Arugula

 30 minutes (including baking time)

Nutritional Information (per serving): Calories: 260 kcal, Protein: 12g, Fat: 7g, Carbohydrates: 40g, Fiber: 4g, Sodium: 310mg

Ingredients (for one serving):
- 1 whole wheat pizza base
- 3 tablespoons unsweetened tomato sauce
- 1 cup sliced fresh mushrooms
- 1 cup fresh arugula
- 2 tablespoons light ricotta cheese

Instructions:
1. Preheat the oven to 200°C (approximately 400°F).
2. Spread the unsweetened tomato sauce evenly over the whole wheat pizza base.
3. Arrange the sliced fresh mushrooms on top of the tomato sauce.
4. Place the pizza in the preheated oven and bake for about 15-18 minutes or until the crust is golden brown and the toppings are cooked.
5. Once baked, remove the pizza from the oven and let it cool for a few minutes.
6. Scatter the fresh arugula over the baked pizza.
7. Dollop teaspoon-sized portions of light ricotta cheese evenly over the arugula.
8. Slice the pizza into portions and serve hot.
9. Enjoy your delicious Pizza with Mushrooms and Arugula!

92. Pizza with Smoked Salmon and Avocado

 25 minutes (including baking time)

Nutritional Information (per serving): Calories: 290 kcal, Protein: 16g, Fat: 14g, Carbohydrates: 26g, Fiber: 4g, Sodium: 320mg

Ingredients (for one serving):

- 1 whole wheat pizza base
- 3 tablespoons unsweetened tomato sauce
- 2 ounces sliced smoked salmon
- 1/2 sliced avocado
- 1/4 thinly sliced red onion

Instructions:

1. Preheat the oven to 200°C (approximately 400°F).
2. Spread the unsweetened tomato sauce evenly over the whole wheat pizza base.
3. Arrange the sliced smoked salmon on top of the tomato sauce.
4. Place the sliced avocado pieces evenly over the smoked salmon.
5. Scatter the thinly sliced red onion over the avocado.
6. Place the pizza in the preheated oven and bake for about 12-15 minutes or until the crust is golden brown.
7. Once baked, remove the pizza from the oven and let it cool for a few minutes.
8. Slice the pizza into portions and serve hot.
9. Enjoy your delicious Pizza with Smoked Salmon and Avocado!

93. Pizza with Tomatoes and Fresh Basil

 20 minutes (including baking time)

Nutritional Information (per serving): Calories: 260 kcal, Protein: 12g, Fat: 10g, Carbohydrates: 30g, Fiber: 3.5g, Sodium: 310mg

Ingredients (for one serving):

- 1 whole wheat pizza base
- 3 tablespoons unsweetened tomato sauce
- 2 sliced tomatoes
- 1/2 cup light mozzarella
- Fresh basil leaves for garnish

Instructions:

1. Preheat the oven to 200°C (approximately 400°F).
2. Spread the unsweetened tomato sauce evenly over the whole wheat pizza base.
3. Arrange the sliced tomatoes on top of the tomato sauce.
4. Sprinkle the light mozzarella evenly over the tomatoes.
5. Place the pizza in the preheated oven and bake for about 12-15 minutes or until the crust is golden brown and the cheese is melted and bubbly.
6. Once baked, remove the pizza from the oven and let it cool for a few minutes.
7. Garnish the pizza with fresh basil leaves before serving.
8. Slice the pizza into portions and serve hot.
9. Enjoy your delicious Pizza with Tomatoes and Fresh Basil!

94. Pizza with Mixed Mushrooms and Caramelized Onions

 25 minutes (including baking time)

Nutritional Information (per serving): Calories: 280 kcal, Protein: 10g, Fat: 9g, Carbohydrates: 40g, Fiber: 4g, Sodium: 310mg

Ingredients (for one serving):
- 1 whole wheat pizza base
- 3 tablespoons unsweetened tomato sauce
- 1 cup mixed mushrooms (portobello, champignon, shiitake), sliced
- 1/2 cup caramelized red onions
- 1/4 cup light gorgonzola cheese, crumbled

Instructions:
1. Preheat the oven to 200°C (approximately 400°F).
2. Spread the unsweetened tomato sauce evenly over the whole wheat pizza base.
3. Arrange the sliced mixed mushrooms and caramelized red onions on top of the tomato sauce.
4. Crumble the light gorgonzola cheese evenly over the mushrooms and onions.
5. Place the pizza in the preheated oven and bake for about 12-15 minutes or until the crust is golden brown and the cheese is melted and bubbly.
6. Once baked, remove the pizza from the oven and let it cool for a few minutes.
7. Slice the pizza into portions and serve hot.
8. Enjoy your delicious Pizza with Mixed Mushrooms and Caramelized Onions!

95. Pizza with Shrimp and Arugula Pesto

 30 minutes (including baking time)

Nutritional Information (per serving): Calories: 270 kcal, Protein: 15g, Fat: 10g, Carbohydrates: 30g, Fiber: 3g, Sodium: 320mg

Ingredients (for one serving):
- 1 whole wheat pizza base
- 3 tablespoons homemade arugula pesto
- 1/2 cup cooked shrimp, peeled and deveined
- 1/4 cup sliced yellow bell peppers
- 1/4 cup crumbled feta cheese

Instructions:
1. Preheat the oven to 200°C (approximately 400°F).
2. Spread the homemade arugula pesto evenly over the whole wheat pizza base.
3. Arrange the cooked shrimp and sliced yellow bell peppers on top of the pesto.
4. Evenly distribute the crumbled feta cheese over the shrimp and peppers.
5. Place the pizza in the preheated oven and bake for about 15-18 minutes or until the crust is golden brown and the cheese is melted and bubbly.
6. Once baked, remove the pizza from the oven and let it cool for a few minutes.
7. Slice the pizza into portions and serve hot.
8. Enjoy your delicious Pizza with Shrimp and Arugula Pesto!

96. Pizza with Mushrooms and Spinach

 25 minutes (including baking time)

Nutritional Information (per serving): Calories: 270 kcal, Protein: 12g, Fat: 8g, Carbohydrates: 38g, Fiber: 4g, Sodium: 330mg

Ingredients (for one serving):
- 1 whole wheat pizza base
- 3 tablespoons unsweetened tomato sauce
- 1/2 cup sliced fresh mushrooms
- 1 cup fresh spinach leaves
- 1/4 cup light ricotta cheese

Instructions:
1. Preheat the oven to 200°C (approximately 400°F).
2. Spread the unsweetened tomato sauce evenly over the whole wheat pizza base.
3. Arrange the sliced fresh mushrooms and fresh spinach leaves on top of the tomato sauce.
4. Evenly distribute the light ricotta cheese over the mushrooms and spinach.
5. Place the pizza in the preheated oven and bake for about 15-18 minutes or until the crust is golden brown and the cheese is melted and bubbly.
6. Once baked, remove the pizza from the oven and let it cool for a few minutes.
7. Slice the pizza into portions and serve hot.
8. Enjoy your delicious Pizza with Mushrooms and Spinach!

CUISINES FROM AROUND THE WORLD

Italian Recipes

97. Spaghetti alla Puttanesca

 25 minutes  1

Nutritional Values (per serving): Calories: approximately 280 kcal, Protein: approximately 9g, Fat: approximately 8g, Carbohydrates: approximately 42g, Fiber: approximately 5g, Sodium: approximately 400mg

Ingredients:
- 100g whole wheat spaghetti
- 200g canned peeled tomatoes
- 2 fillets of anchovies in oil
- 1 tablespoon capers, rinsed
- 1/6 cup pitted and sliced black olives
- 1 clove garlic, finely chopped
- 1/2 fresh chili pepper, finely chopped (optional)
- 1 tablespoon finely chopped fresh parsley
- Extra virgin olive oil
- Salt and pepper to taste

Instructions:
1. Bring a pot of salted water to a boil and cook the whole wheat spaghetti according to package instructions. When al dente, drain them, reserving some cooking water.
2. In a pan, heat some extra virgin olive oil over medium heat. Add the chopped garlic and fresh chili pepper, if using. Sauté for about 1 minute until the garlic turns golden and fragrant.
3. Add the canned peeled tomatoes to the pan, lightly crushing them with a fork. Cook over medium-low heat for 10-15 minutes, stirring occasionally, until the sauce thickens.
4. Add the roughly chopped anchovies in oil, capers, and black olives to the sauce. Mix well and cook for another 5-7 minutes.
5. Add the spaghetti to the pan with the puttanesca sauce and gently toss until the spaghetti are well coated with the sauce. If needed, add some reserved spaghetti cooking water to achieve the desired consistency.
6. Continue to cook for another 2-3 minutes until the spaghetti are well heated through and have absorbed the flavors of the sauce.
7. Before serving, sprinkle the spaghetti with finely chopped fresh parsley and adjust the seasoning with salt and pepper to your taste.
8. Serve the hot and flavorful Spaghetti alla Puttanesca, garnishing with extra finely chopped fresh parsley if desired. Enjoy!

Chicken Cacciatore

98. Chicken Cacciatore

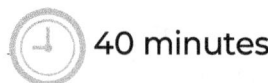 40 minutes    1

Nutritional Values (per serving): Calories: approximately 280 kcal, Protein: approximately 30g, Fat: approximately 10g, Carbohydrates: approximately 10g, Fiber: approximately 4g, Sodium: approximately 320mg

Ingredients:
- 1 chicken breast (about 150g)
- 100g canned peeled tomatoes
- 1/4 onion, chopped
- 1 carrot, sliced
- 1 stalk celery, chopped
- 1/8 cup dry white wine
- 1 sprig fresh rosemary
- 1 tablespoon extra virgin olive oil
- Salt and pepper to taste

Instructions:
1. In a large non-stick skillet, heat the extra virgin olive oil over medium-high heat.
2. Add the chicken breast to the skillet and brown it on both sides until golden, about 5-7 minutes per side. Transfer the chicken to a plate and set aside.
3. In the same skillet, add the chopped onion, carrot, and celery. Cook for about 5 minutes or until the vegetables begin to soften.
4. Add the canned peeled tomatoes, white wine, and sprig of rosemary to the skillet. Stir well and bring to a boil.
5. Reduce the heat to medium-low and return the chicken breast to the skillet along with the tomato sauce. Cover the skillet with a lid and let it cook for about 20-25 minutes, stirring occasionally, until the chicken is fully cooked and the sauce has slightly thickened.
6. Ensure the chicken is cooked through and the sauce has reached a thick and flavorful consistency. Adjust the seasoning with salt and pepper to your personal taste.
7. Once the chicken cacciatore is ready, remove the rosemary sprig and serve the dish hot.
8. Serve the Chicken Cacciatore with side dishes such as basmati rice, roasted potatoes, or grilled vegetables. Enjoy!

99. Eggplant Parmigiana Light

Nutritional Values (per serving): Calories: about 200-250 kcal, Fat: about 10-12g, Carbohydrates: about 15-20g, Protein: about 10-12, Fiber: about 5-7g, Sodium: varies depending on the amount of added salt.

Ingredients:
- 2 medium eggplants
- 400g peeled tomatoes
- 200g light mozzarella
- 50g grated light Parmesan cheese
- Extra virgin olive oil
- Salt
- Pepper
- Fresh basil

Instructions:
1. Preheat the oven to 180°C (356°F).
2. Slice the eggplants thinly, about 1/2 cm thick. Place them on a baking tray, sprinkle some salt on both sides, and let them sit for about 15 minutes to remove bitterness.
3. After 15 minutes, pat the eggplant slices dry with paper towels to remove excess moisture.
4. In a non-stick pan, heat a bit of extra virgin olive oil over medium heat and cook the eggplant slices on both sides until they become soft and lightly golden. They should not be fried, just lightly golden to soften. Place the cooked slices on a plate lined with paper towels to remove excess oil.
5. In a pot, heat the peeled tomatoes with a pinch of salt and pepper and a few fresh basil leaves. Cook for about 10-15 minutes over medium-low heat, mashing the tomatoes with a fork to achieve a sauce-like consistency.
6. Slice the mozzarella thinly.
7. Take an oven dish and start assembling the dish. Pour some tomato sauce on the bottom, then add a layer of eggplant slices, followed by slices of mozzarella and grated Parmesan cheese. Repeat the layers until all ingredients are used up, finishing with a final layer of tomato sauce and grated Parmesan cheese.
8. Place the dish in the preheated oven and bake for about 25-30 minutes, until the cheese is golden and the surface of the Parmigiana is crispy.
9. Once cooked, let the Eggplant Parmigiana rest for a few minutes before serving. Garnish with fresh basil leaves and serve hot.

100. Whole Wheat Pasta with Tomato and Basil

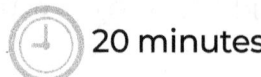 20 minutes

Nutritional Values (per serving): Calories: about 300 kcal, Protein: about 8g, Fat: about 10g, Carbohydrates: about 45g, Fiber: about 6g, Sodium: about 200mg

Ingredients:
- 100g whole wheat pasta
- 2 fresh tomatoes, diced
- 1 clove of garlic, minced
- 1/2 bunch of fresh basil, chopped
- 1 1/2 tablespoons of extra virgin olive oil
- Salt and pepper to taste

Instructions:
1. Bring a pot of salted water to a boil and cook the whole wheat pasta according to the package instructions until al dente. Drain the pasta, reserving some cooking water.
2. While the pasta cooks, heat the olive oil in a pan over medium heat. Add the minced garlic and sauté until golden, being careful not to burn it.
3. Add the diced fresh tomatoes to the pan with the garlic. Cook for about 8-10 minutes, stirring occasionally, until the tomatoes soften and release their juices.
4. When the tomatoes are soft, add half of the chopped basil to the pan. Continue to cook for another 2-3 minutes to allow the basil to release its aroma.
5. Add the drained pasta to the pan with the tomato and basil sauce. Mix well to evenly coat the pasta. If necessary, add some pasta cooking water to reach the desired consistency.
6. Season with salt and pepper to taste.
7. Serve the Whole Wheat Pasta with Tomato and Basil hot, garnished with the remaining fresh basil as a finishing touch.

Enjoy your meal!

101. Caprese Salad

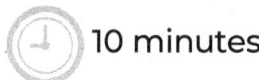 10 minutes

Nutritional Values (per serving): Calories: about 200 kcal, Protein: about 10g, Fat: about 15g, Carbohydrates: about 5g, Fiber: about 2g, Sodium: about 150mg

Ingredients:
- 2 ripe tomatoes
- 100g buffalo mozzarella
- Fresh basil leaves, as needed
- 1 tablespoon extra virgin olive oil
- 1 tablespoon balsamic vinegar
- Salt and pepper to taste

Instructions:
1. Slice the tomatoes and buffalo mozzarella into thin slices.
2. Alternately arrange the tomato and mozzarella slices on a serving plate, creating a mosaic pattern.
3. Add some fresh basil leaves between the tomatoes and mozzarella.
4. Drizzle the salad with a drizzle of extra virgin olive oil and balsamic vinegar.
5. Season with salt and pepper according to your taste.
6. Serve immediately to enjoy the freshness of the Caprese Salad.

102. Bruschetta with Cherry Tomatoes and Basil

 15 minutes  1

Nutritional Values (per serving): Calories: about 180 kcal, Protein: about 4g, Fat: about 8g, Carbohydrates: about 22g, Fiber: about 3g, Sodium: about 160mg

Ingredients:
- 2 slices of whole wheat bread
- 100g cherry tomatoes
- 1 garlic clove
- Fresh basil leaves, as needed
- 1 tablespoon extra virgin olive oil
- Salt and pepper to taste

Instructions:
1. Toast the slices of whole wheat bread until crispy.
2. Cut the cherry tomatoes in half.
3. Rub the garlic clove over the toasted bread slices to add a subtle aroma.
4. Place the halved cherry tomatoes on the toasted bread slices.
5. Add some fresh basil leaves on top of the cherry tomatoes.
6. Drizzle the bruschetta with a drizzle of extra virgin olive oil.
7. Season with salt and pepper according to your taste.
8. Serve the bruschetta immediately to enjoy the fresh and aromatic flavors.

103. Whole Wheat Linguine with Avocado Sauce

 15 minutes

Nutritional Values (per serving):

Nutritions: Calories: about 270 kcal, Protein: about 6g, Fat: about 14g, Carbohydrates: about 30g, Fiber: about 5g, Sodium: about 170mg

Ingredients:
- 100g whole wheat linguine
- 1/2 ripe avocado
- 1 garlic clove
- Juice of 1/2 lemon
- 1 tablespoon extra virgin olive oil
- A handful of fresh parsley
- Salt and pepper to taste

Instructions:
1. In a pot, bring a sufficient amount of salted water to a boil. Add the whole wheat linguine and cook according to the package instructions until al dente. Drain them and set aside.
2. Meanwhile, prepare the avocado sauce. In a blender or food processor, add the flesh of the ripe avocado, peeled garlic clove, lemon juice, extra virgin olive oil, and fresh parsley. Blend until you get a creamy and homogeneous sauce. Season with salt and pepper according to your taste.
3. Pour the avocado sauce over the cooked whole wheat linguine and gently toss until evenly coated.
4. Serve the Whole Wheat Linguine with Avocado Sauce in a bowl, garnishing with fresh parsley leaves and a sprinkle of freshly ground black pepper, if desired.

French Recipes

104. Ratatouille

Nutritional Values (per approximate serving): Calories: about 120 kcal, Protein: 2g, Carbohydrates: 14g, Fat: 7g, Fiber: 4g, Sodium: 180mg

Ingredients:
- 1 eggplant
- 2 zucchinis
- 1 red bell pepper
- 2 tomatoes
- 1 onion
- 2 cloves of garlic
- 2 tablespoons olive oil
- 1 tablespoon chopped fresh thyme
- Salt and pepper to taste

Instructions:
1. Slice all the vegetables: eggplant, zucchinis, bell pepper, and tomatoes. Finely chop the onion and garlic.
2. In a large skillet, heat the olive oil over medium heat. Add the chopped onion and garlic and sauté until golden and soft, about 3-4 minutes.
3. Add the sliced vegetables (eggplant, zucchinis, bell pepper, and tomatoes) to the skillet with the sautéed onion and garlic. Mix well to evenly distribute the oil and spices.
4. Cook the vegetables over medium heat, stirring occasionally, until they become tender but not too mushy, about 20-25 minutes.
5. Once the vegetables are cooked, add the chopped fresh thyme and adjust salt and pepper to taste. Mix well to incorporate the flavors.
6. Once ready, serve the Ratatouille warm.

105. Coq au Vin (Chicken in Wine)

 About 1 hour and 30 minutes  1

Nutritional Values (per serving): Calories: about 250 kcal, Protein: about 20g, Carbohydrates: about 10g, Fat: about 12g, Fiber: about 2g, Sodium: about 200mg

Ingredients:
- 1 chicken thigh
- 25g diced lean bacon
- 1/4 onion
- 1/2 carrot
- 50g mushrooms
- 62.5ml red wine
- 125ml vegetable broth
- 1 sprig fresh thyme
- 1 bay leaf
- 1/2 tablespoon olive oil
- Salt and pepper to taste

Instructions:
1. In a large pot, heat the olive oil over medium heat. Add the diced bacon and fry until golden and crispy.
2. Add the chicken thigh to the pot and brown it on both sides until golden, about 5 minutes per side.
3. Add the sliced onion, diced carrot, and sliced mushrooms to the pot. Continue to cook for another 5 minutes, stirring occasionally.
4. Pour the red wine into the pot and let it evaporate, about 2-3 minutes.
5. Add the vegetable broth to cover the ingredients in the pot. Also, add the fresh thyme and bay leaf. Bring it to a boil, then reduce the heat and let it simmer for about 1 hour or until the chicken is tender.
6. Once the chicken is cooked, taste the sauce and adjust salt and pepper to your liking.
7. Serve the Coq au Vin hot, perhaps accompanied by some crusty bread to dip into the flavorful sauce.

106. Bouillabaisse (Fish Soup)

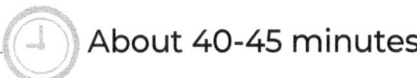
About 40-45 minutes

Nutritional Values (per serving): Calories: about 220 kcal, Protein: about 20g, Carbohydrates: about 15g, Fat: about 8g, Fiber: about 3g, Sodium: about 170mg

Ingredients:
- 100g mixed fish (cod, sea bream, shrimp)
- 1 tomato
- 1/2 potato
- 1/4 onion
- 1 clove of garlic
- 1/2 tablespoon chopped fresh parsley
- 250ml fish broth
- A pinch of saffron
- 1 tablespoon olive oil
- Salt and pepper to taste

Instructions:
1. In a large pot, heat the olive oil over medium heat. Add the chopped onion and crushed garlic and sauté until golden and soft.
2. Add the diced tomato to the pot and cook until a thick sauce forms.
3. Add the peeled and diced potato to the pot, then pour in the fish broth. Bring it to a boil, then reduce the heat and let it simmer until the potatoes are tender, about 15-20 minutes.
4. Add the mixed fish to the pot along with the chopped fresh parsley and saffron. Simmer for another 15-20 minutes until the fish is cooked and tender.
5. Taste the bouillabaisse and adjust salt and pepper according to your taste.
6. Serve the bouillabaisse hot, accompanied by toasted bread slices.

107. Cassoulet

About 1 hour and 45 minutes

Nutritional Values (per serving): Calories: about 320 kcal, Protein: about 20g, Carbohydrates: about 25g, Fat: about 15g, Fiber: about 6g, Sodium: about 250mg

Ingredients:
- 100g white beans
- 1/2 sausage
- 50g bacon
- 1 chicken thigh
- 1/4 onion
- 1 clove of garlic
- 200ml chicken broth
- 100g diced tomatoes
- 1 tablespoon chopped fresh parsley
- 1 tablespoon olive oil
- Salt and pepper to taste

Instructions:
1. In a large pot, heat olive oil over medium heat. Add diced bacon and fry until golden and crispy.
2. Add chopped onion and crushed garlic to the pot and sauté until softened.
3. Add sausage and chicken thigh to the pot and brown on both sides.
4. Add drained white beans, diced tomatoes, and chicken broth to the pot. Mix well.
5. Bring the cassoulet to a boil, then reduce heat and let simmer for about 1 hour and 30 minutes, until the cassoulet is thick and flavorful, and the chicken is cooked.
6. Taste the cassoulet and adjust salt and pepper to your liking.
7. Serve the cassoulet hot, sprinkled with plenty of chopped fresh parsley.

108. Quiche with Vegetables

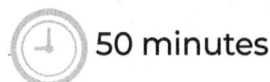 50 minutes  1

Nutritional Values (per serving): Calories: about 220 kcal, Protein: about 9g, Carbohydrates: about 15g, Fat: about 13g, Fiber: about 2g, Sodium: about 190mg

Ingredients:
- 1/4 puff pastry
- 1 egg
- 50ml skim milk
- 50g fresh spinach
- 37.5g cherry tomatoes
- 1/4 onion
- 12.5g grated cheese
- 1/2 tablespoon olive oil
- Salt and pepper to taste

Instructions:
1. Preheat the oven to 180°C (350°F). Line a quiche pan with puff pastry and prick the bottom with a fork. Set aside.
2. In a pan, heat olive oil over medium heat. Add chopped onion and lightly sauté.
3. Add washed and squeezed fresh spinach to the pan and cook until slightly wilted. Remove from heat and let cool.
4. In a bowl, beat the egg with milk, grated cheese, salt, and pepper.
5. Pour the spinach mixture over the puff pastry base in the quiche pan.
6. Pour the beaten egg mixture on top.
7. Cut the cherry tomatoes in half and arrange them on the surface of the quiche.
8. Bake the quiche in the preheated oven for about 30-35 minutes or until the surface is golden and the center is cooked.
9. Once cooked, remove the quiche from the oven and let it cool slightly before slicing and serving.

109. Beef Bourguignon

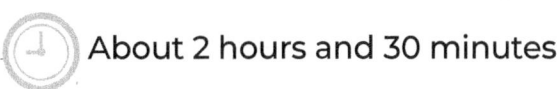 About 2 hours and 30 minutes

Nutritional Values (per serving): Calories: about 280 kcal, Protein: about 25g, Carbohydrates: about 18g, Fat: about 10g, Fiber: about 4g, Sodium: about 220mg

Ingredients:
- 125g beef (e.g., chuck or sirloin)
- 62.5ml red wine
- 1 onion
- 1 carrot
- 1 potato
- 1.5 cloves of garlic
- 250ml beef broth
- 1 sprig fresh thyme
- 1 bay leaf
- 1 tablespoon olive oil
- Salt and pepper to taste

Instructions:
1. Cut the piece of beef into uniform-sized pieces.
2. In a large pot, heat olive oil over medium-high heat. Add the beef and brown it on all sides until well browned. Remove the beef from the pot and set it aside.
3. Meanwhile, slice the onion, carrot, and potato. Chop the garlic.
4. In the same pot, add the onion and carrot and sauté for a few minutes until softened.
5. Pour the red wine into the pot and let the alcohol evaporate.
6. Add the potato, chopped garlic, fresh thyme, and bay leaf. Also, add the browned beef.
7. Pour the beef broth into the pot until the meat and vegetables are completely covered.
8. Bring it to a boil, then reduce the heat and let it simmer over low heat for about 2 hours, or until the meat is tender and the sauce is thick and aromatic. During cooking, stir occasionally and add some water if necessary to prevent the bottom from drying out too much.
9. Once the Beef Bourguignon is ready, remove the bay leaf and fresh thyme. Taste and adjust salt and pepper if necessary.
10. 1Serve the Beef Bourguignon hot, accompanied by crusty bread or roasted potatoes, if desired.

Greek Recipes

110. Chicken Souvlaki with Tzatziki

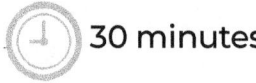 30 minutes

Nutritional Values (per serving): Calories: about 250 kcal, Protein: about 20g, Fat: about 10g, Carbohydrates: about 15g, Fiber: about 1g, Sodium: about 220mg

Ingredients:
- 125g chicken breast
- 1/2 lemon
- 1 clove garlic
- 1/2 teaspoon oregano
- 62.5g low-fat Greek yogurt
- 1/4 cucumber
- Some fresh parsley
- 1 teaspoon olive oil
- Salt and pepper to taste

Instructions:
1. Cut the chicken breast into cubes and place them in a bowl.
2. Add the juice of half a lemon, minced garlic, oregano, salt, and pepper to the chicken cubes. Mix well to ensure the chicken is well-marinated. Let it marinate for at least 15-20 minutes.
3. Thread the marinated chicken cubes onto a skewer.
4. Heat a grill or non-stick pan and lightly brush with olive oil.
5. Grill the chicken skewers on the grill or in the pan until golden brown and fully cooked, turning occasionally for even cooking.
6. Meanwhile, prepare the tzatziki sauce. Grate the cucumber and squeeze out excess water. Mix the low-fat Greek yogurt with the grated cucumber, minced garlic, chopped fresh parsley, remaining lemon juice, salt, and pepper.
7. Once the chicken skewers are ready, serve them hot with the prepared tzatziki sauce.
8. Enjoy your Chicken Souvlaki with Tzatziki!

111. Greek Salad

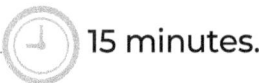 15 minutes.

Nutritional Values (per serving): Calories: about 180 kcal, Protein: about 5g, Fat: about 12g, Carbohydrates: about 12g, Fiber: about 3g, Sodium: about 320mg

Ingredients (per serving):
- 1 medium tomato
- 1/2 cucumber
- 4-5 black olives
- 1/4 red onion
- Fresh chili pepper to taste
- 1 teaspoon dried oregano
- 30g light feta cheese
- 1 tablespoon olive oil
- 1 tablespoon red wine vinegar
- Salt and pepper to taste

Instructions:
1. Dice the tomato and cucumber and place them in a bowl.
2. Slice the red onion and chili pepper, and add them to the bowl.
3. Add the pitted black olives.
4. Crumble the feta cheese and add it to the bowl along with the oregano.
5. Dress the salad with olive oil and red wine vinegar.
6. Season with salt and pepper to taste.
7. Mix all the ingredients well and serve the fresh and fragrant Greek salad.
8. These quantities and nutritional values are approximate and may vary slightly depending on the exact sizes of the ingredients used. Enjoy your meal!

112. Melitzanosalata

 45 minutes.

Nutritional Values (per serving): Calories: about 120 kcal, Protein: about 2g, Fat: about 10g, Carbohydrates: about 8g, Fiber: about 4g, Sodium: about 200mg

Ingredients (per serving):
- 1 medium eggplant
- 1 clove garlic
- Juice of 1/2 lemon
- 1 tablespoon chopped fresh parsley
- 1 tablespoon olive oil
- Salt and pepper to taste

Instructions:
1. Grill the whole eggplant until the skin is well-charred and the flesh is soft. This process may take about 30-40 minutes, turning the eggplant occasionally to ensure even cooking.
2. Once cooked, allow the eggplant to cool slightly, then peel it and mash the flesh with a fork or blender.
3. Transfer the eggplant pulp to a bowl and add finely chopped garlic.
4. Add lemon juice, chopped fresh parsley, and olive oil.
5. Season with salt and pepper to taste and mix all the ingredients well until smooth and homogeneous.
6. Serve the melitzanosalata as an appetizer or side dish, garnished perhaps with a drizzle of olive oil and some fresh parsley leaves.

113. Spanakopita

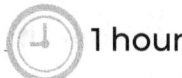 1 hour

Nutritions: Calories: about 180 kcal, Protein: about 7g, Fat: about 10g, Carbohydrates: about 15g, Fiber: about 2g, Sodium: about 230mg

Ingredients:
- 200g fresh spinach
- 1 onion
- A bunch of fresh parsley
- Some fresh mint leaves
- 100g light feta cheese
- 2 eggs
- 2 tablespoons olive oil
- Phyllo pastry sheets

Instructions:
1. Finely chop the onion and sauté it with a tablespoon of olive oil in a large skillet until translucent.
2. Add the washed and drained spinach to the skillet and cook until wilted and most of the water is released.
3. Chop the fresh parsley and mint and add them to the spinach. Mix well.
4. Beat the eggs in a bowl and add them to the spinach mixture. Also, add the crumbled feta cheese. Mix all ingredients well.
5. Lightly brush a sheet of phyllo pastry with olive oil and layer another sheet on top of it. Add some of the spinach filling along the edge and fold the phyllo pastry sheet in half to form a triangle. Continue this process until all ingredients are used.
6. Arrange the phyllo pastry triangles on a baking sheet lined with parchment paper and brush the surface with a little olive oil.
7. Bake in a preheated oven at 180°C (350°F) for about 20-25 minutes or until golden and crispy.
8. Once cooked, serve your delicious spanakopita hot or at room temperature.
9. These nutritional values and preparation times are approximate and may vary slightly depending on the exact ingredients used and cooking techniques. Enjoy your meal!

114. Fasolada (Bean Soup)

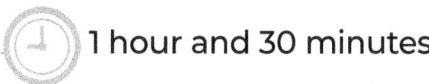 1 hour and 30 minutes

Nutritional Values (per serving): Calories: about 200 kcal, Protein: 6g, Fat: 5g, Carbohydrates: 30g, Fiber: 5g, Sodium: 180mg

Ingredients:
- 200g cannellini beans
- 2 carrots, diced
- 2 celery stalks, chopped
- 2 tomatoes, diced
- 1 onion, chopped
- 2 cloves garlic, minced
- A bunch of fresh parsley, chopped
- 1 teaspoon dried oregano
- 2 tablespoons olive oil
- Salt and pepper to taste

Instructions:
1. In a large pot, heat olive oil over medium heat. Add chopped onion, diced carrots, and chopped celery. Sauté until the vegetables become tender, stirring occasionally.
2. Add minced garlic cloves to the pot and cook for about a minute until fragrant.
3. Add diced tomatoes and cook for another 5 minutes, stirring occasionally.
4. Pour cooked cannellini beans into the pot along with the vegetables. Also, add chopped parsley and dried oregano. Mix well.
5. Add enough water to cover all the ingredients in the pot. Bring it to a boil, then reduce the heat and let it simmer for about 1 hour, or until the beans become soft and the soup slightly thickens.
6. Taste the fasolada and adjust salt and pepper according to your personal taste.
7. Once the bean soup reaches the desired consistency, remove it from the heat and serve hot.

115. Chickpea Tzatziki

Ingredients:
- 200g canned chickpeas, drained and rinsed
- 100g Greek yogurt (or vegan yogurt)
- 1 cucumber
- 2 cloves garlic
- Juice of 1/2 lemon
- 2 tablespoons olive oil
- Salt and pepper to taste
- Fresh mint leaves

Instructions:
1. In a bowl, lightly mash the chickpeas with a fork to achieve a creamier consistency.
2. Finely chop the cucumber and garlic.
3. Add Greek yogurt (or vegan yogurt), chopped cucumber, minced garlic, lemon juice, and olive oil to the same bowl.
4. Season with a pinch of salt and pepper and some chopped fresh mint leaves for flavor.
5. Mix all ingredients well until you get a homogeneous mixture.
6. Taste and adjust salt and pepper according to your personal preference.
7. Store the chickpea tzatziki in the refrigerator until ready to serve.
8. Serve the chickpea tzatziki as a dip for fresh vegetables or as a side dish for meat or fish dishes.

Chinese Recipes

116. Vegetable Fried Rice

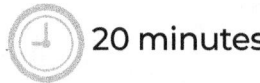 20 minutes

Nutritional Values (per serving): Calories: about 250 kcal, Protein: about 10g, Fat: about 5g, Carbohydrates: about 40g, Fiber: about 5g, Sodium: 250mg

Ingredients:
- 100g cooked and cooled brown rice
- 2 egg whites
- 100g mixed vegetables (carrots, peas, Chinese cabbage)
- 1 teaspoon sesame oil
- Low-sodium soy sauce (to be used moderately)

Instructions:
1. In a non-stick pan, heat sesame oil over medium heat.
2. Add diced mixed vegetables to the pan and stir-fry until tender.
3. Add the cooked and cooled brown rice to the pan with the vegetables and mix well.
4. Lightly beat the egg whites and pour them over the rice and vegetable mixture in the pan.
5. Stir continuously until the egg whites solidify and mix evenly with the rice and vegetables.
6. Add low-sodium soy sauce moderately and mix well to flavor the fried rice.
7. Continue to cook for a few minutes, stirring occasionally, until everything is well heated.
8. Serve the hot vegetable fried rice as a light and tasty main dish.

117. Chicken and Corn Soup:

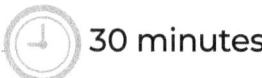 30 minutes

Nutritional Values (per serving): Calories: about 180 kcal, Protein: about 15g, Carbohydrates: about 20g, Fat: about 4g, Fiber: about 3g, Sodium: 200mg

Ingredients:
- 100g chicken breast
- 50g canned corn
- 250ml low-sodium vegetable broth
- 1/4 onion
- 1 clove garlic
- 1 cm fresh ginger
- Fresh parsley
- Black pepper

Instructions:
1. In a pot, bring the vegetable broth to a boil along with chopped onion, crushed garlic, and grated fresh ginger.
2. Once the broth starts boiling, add the whole chicken breast and let it cook until fully cooked through, about 15-20 minutes.
3. When the chicken breast is cooked, remove it from the pot and dice it.
4. Add the canned corn to the pot along with the diced chicken. Let it cook for another 10 minutes over medium heat.
5. Add chopped fresh parsley and freshly ground black pepper. Mix well.
6. Taste the soup and adjust the seasoning with salt and pepper, if necessary.
7. Serve the hot chicken and corn soup, optionally garnished with some additional fresh parsley.

118. Cabbage and Carrot Salad:

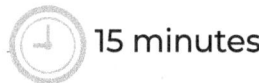 15 minutes

Nutritional Values (per serving): Calories: about 120 kcal, Protein: about 2g, Carbohydrates: about 8g, Fat: about 9g, Fiber: about 4g, Sodium: 150mg

Ingredients:
- 100g Chinese cabbage
- 50g carrots
- 1 tablespoon rice vinegar
- 1 tablespoon sesame oil
- 1 cm grated fresh ginger
- 1 tablespoon toasted sesame seeds

Instructions:
1. Finely shred the Chinese cabbage and grate the carrots.
2. In a large bowl, toss the cabbage and carrots with rice vinegar, sesame oil, and grated ginger.
3. Sprinkle with toasted sesame seeds before serving.
4. Mix well and ensure the salad is evenly dressed.
5. Serve the cabbage and carrot salad as a light and healthy side dish.

119. Steamed Orange Chicken

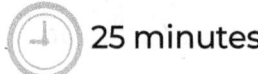 25 minutes

Nutritional Values (per serving): Calories: about 200 kcal, Protein: about 25g, Carbohydrates: about 10g, Fat: about 5g, Fiber: about 2g, Sodium: 220mg

Ingredients:
- 200g chicken breast
- Fresh juice of 2 oranges
- Zest of 1 orange
- 2 cloves garlic, minced
- 1 cm fresh ginger, grated
- 1 tablespoon low-sodium soy sauce
- 1 teaspoon cornstarch

Instructions:
1. Slice the chicken breast into thin strips.
2. In a bowl, mix orange juice, grated orange zest, minced garlic, grated ginger, soy sauce, and cornstarch.
3. Place the chicken in the marinade and let it marinate for at least 15 minutes.
4. Transfer the chicken and marinade to a steamer and steam for about 15 minutes or until the chicken is fully cooked.
5. Serve the steamed orange chicken with a splash of fresh orange juice and a sprinkle of grated orange zest. Serve with your choice of sides.

Enjoy your meal!

120. Stir-Fried Tofu with Vegetables

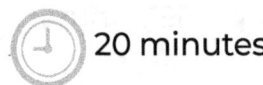 20 minutes

Nutritional Values (per serving): Calories: about 180 kcal, Protein: about 10g, Carbohydrates: about 10g, Fat: about 10g, Fiber: about 5g, Sodium: 200mg

Ingredients:
- 150g tofu
- 100g broccoli
- 1 bell pepper
- 1/2 onion
- 2 tablespoons low-sodium soy sauce
- 2 cloves garlic, minced
- 1 tablespoon sesame oil

Instructions:
1. Cut the tofu into cubes and the vegetables into pieces.
2. In a non-stick skillet, heat a little sesame oil and sauté the minced garlic until golden.
3. Add the vegetables (broccoli, bell pepper, and onion) to the skillet and stir-fry until tender.
4. Add the tofu to the skillet and pour in the soy sauce. Cook for another 5-7 minutes, stirring occasionally, until the tofu is heated through and the vegetables are cooked to your liking.
5. Serve the stir-fried tofu with vegetables hot, optionally garnished with toasted sesame seeds.

121. Steamed Chinese Dumplings with Spinach and Mushroom Filling

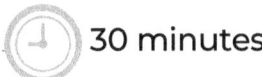 30 minutes

Nutritional Values (per serving): Calories: about 220 kcal, Protein: about 8g, Carbohydrates: about 40g, Fat: about 2g, Fiber: about 3g, Sodium: 180mg

Ingredients:
- 200g Chinese dumpling wrappers
- 100g fresh spinach
- 100g shiitake mushrooms
- 2 cloves garlic, minced
- 1 piece fresh ginger, grated
- 2 tablespoons low-sodium soy sauce

Instructions:
1. Finely chop the fresh spinach and shiitake mushrooms.
2. In a skillet, heat some oil and sauté the minced garlic and grated ginger until golden and fragrant.
3. Add the chopped spinach and shiitake mushrooms to the skillet and sauté until tender.
4. Add the low-sodium soy sauce to the skillet and mix well. Cook for a few more minutes, then remove from heat and let the filling cool.
5. Prepare the Chinese dumplings by placing a spoonful of filling in the center of each dumpling wrapper. Seal the edges tightly by pressing them with your fingers or using a fork.
6. Prepare the steam in the pot and steam the dumplings for about 8-10 minutes, until the wrapper becomes translucent and the filling is hot.
7. Serve the steamed Chinese dumplings hot, optionally accompanied by an additional low-sodium soy sauce dip or a sauce of your choice.

122. Sautéed Zucchini Noodles with Chicken and Soy Sauce

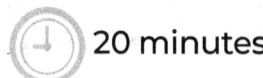 20 minutes

Nutritional Values (per serving): Calories: about 190 kcal, Protein: about 20g, Carbohydrates: about 6g, Fat: about 8g, Fiber: about 3g, Sodium: 210mg

Ingredients:
- 2 zucchinis
- 200g chicken breast, thinly sliced
- 2 cloves garlic, minced
- 2 tablespoons low-sodium soy sauce
- 1 tablespoon sesame oil

Instructions:
1. Using a vegetable peeler, cut the zucchinis into noodles or use a spiralizer to create zucchini noodles. Set aside.
2. In a non-stick skillet, heat sesame oil over medium heat. Add minced garlic and sauté until golden and fragrant.
3. Add the sliced chicken breast to the skillet and cook until well browned on all sides.
4. Add the zucchini noodles to the skillet and pour in the low-sodium soy sauce. Mix well.
5. Sauté everything in the skillet for about 3-5 minutes, or until the zucchini is tender but still crisp and the chicken is fully cooked.
6. Ensure that the sauce is well distributed and all ingredients are heated through.
7. Serve the sautéed zucchini noodles with chicken and soy sauce hot, optionally garnishing with a sprinkle of fresh chili or toasted sesame seeds.

123. Peking Duck with Vegetables

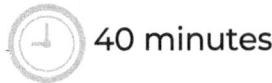 40 minutes

Nutritional Values (per serving): Calories: about 250 kcal, Protein: about 20g, Carbohydrates: about 10g, Fat: about 15g, Fiber: about 4g, Sodium: 220mg

Ingredients:
- 1 duck breast
- 1 Chinese cabbage
- 2 carrots
- 1 bell pepper
- 1 onion
- 4 tablespoons unsweetened plum sauce
- 2 cm ginger root, minced
- Olive oil

Instructions:
1. Preheat the grill to medium-high heat. Grill the duck breast until the skin is crispy and the meat is cooked through. Once cooked, set aside and let it rest.
2. Meanwhile, prepare the vegetables. Julienne the Chinese cabbage, carrots, and bell pepper. Finely chop the onion.
3. In a large skillet, heat some olive oil over medium heat. Add the minced onion and minced ginger and sauté until golden and fragrant.
4. Add the julienned vegetables to the skillet and stir-fry until tender but still crisp.
5. Pour the unsweetened plum sauce over the vegetables and mix well to evenly distribute the sauce.
6. Slice the duck breast into thin slices and serve it over the sautéed vegetables.
7. Serve the Peking duck with vegetables hot, perhaps accompanied by white rice or noodles.

Japanese Recipes

124. Preparation of Sushi Rice

Ingredients:
- Sushi rice (preferably Japanese variety like Koshihikari)
- Rice vinegar
- Sugar
- Salt

Instructions:
1. Rinse the Rice: Place the rice in a bowl and cover it with cold water. Gently agitate the rice with your hands to release the starch. Pour off the cloudy water and repeat the process until the water remains relatively clear.
2. Drain the Rice: After rinsing, drain the rice well in a colander to remove excess water.
3. Cooking the Rice: Transfer the rice to a pot and add water in a 1:1 ratio of rice to water. Cover the pot with a lid and bring the water to a boil. Once boiling, reduce the heat and let it simmer for about 15-20 minutes, or until the rice absorbs all the water.
4. Resting the Rice: Turn off the heat and let the rice rest covered for another 10-15 minutes. During this time, the rice will finish cooking and absorb any remaining moisture.
5. Preparing the Seasoning: In a small pot, mix rice vinegar, sugar, and salt. Heat over low heat until the sugar and salt are completely dissolved.
6. Season the Rice: Transfer the cooked rice to a large wooden or glass bowl. Pour the prepared seasoning over the rice and gently mix using a wooden spatula. Make sure to evenly distribute the seasoning over the rice.
7. Cooling the Rice: Fan the seasoned rice while gently mixing. This process will help cool the rice without making it too cold.

125. Vegetarian Sushi Rolls:

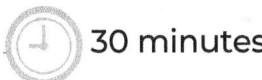 30 minutes

Nutritional Values (per single serving): Calories: about 180 kcal, Protein: about 5g, Carbohydrates: about 30g, Fat: about 5g, Fiber: about 3g, Sodium: 200mg

Ingredients:
- 2 nori seaweed sheets
- 1/2 cup sushi rice
- 1/2 avocado
- 1/4 cucumber
- 1/2 carrot
- 1/4 bell pepper
- 50g tofu
- Low-sodium soy sauce, for serving

Instructions:
1. Prepare the sushi rice following the instructions on the package. Allow it to cool slightly.
2. Slice the avocado, cucumber, carrot, bell pepper, and tofu into thin strips.
3. Lay a sheet of nori seaweed on a flat surface. Spread the sushi rice evenly over the bottom half of the sheet.
4. Arrange strips of avocado, cucumber, carrot, bell pepper, and tofu on top of the rice.
5. Roll the nori seaweed tightly around the filling, using a bamboo mat if necessary.
6. Once rolled, seal the edge of the nori seaweed with a little water to keep it closed.
7. Cut the sushi roll into evenly sized slices using a sharp knife.
8. Arrange the sushi rolls on a serving plate and serve with low-sodium soy sauce for dipping.

126. Sauteed Edamame

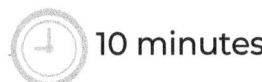 10 minutes

Nutritional values (per serving): Calories: about 120 kcal, Protein: about 10g, Carbohydrates: about 10g, Fat: about 5g, Fiber: about 5g, Sodium: 280mg, Badge: Vegan

Operational Instructions:
1. Blanch the edamame in boiling water for a few minutes, then sauté them in a pan with olive oil and sea salt until lightly golden. Serve hot.

127. Yakitori Chicken with Reduced Teriyaki Sauce

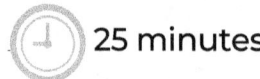 25 minutes

Nutritional Values (per single serving): Calories: about 190 kcal, Protein: about 25g, Carbohydrates: about 8g, Fat: about 5g, Fiber: about 1g, Sodium: 180mg

Ingredients:
- 1 chicken breast
- 2 tablespoons low-sodium teriyaki sauce
- 1 clove garlic, finely chopped
- 1 teaspoon freshly grated ginger
- 1 tablespoon soy sauce
- Juice of 1/2 lemon

Instructions:
1. Cut the chicken breast into pieces and thread them onto skewers.
2. Heat a grill and cook the chicken skewers until fully cooked, turning them occasionally and brushing them with teriyaki sauce during cooking.
3. Meanwhile, prepare the reduced teriyaki sauce. In a saucepan, mix the chopped garlic, grated ginger, soy sauce, and lemon juice. Bring to a boil, then reduce the heat and simmer until the sauce has reduced to a thick consistency, stirring occasionally.
4. Once the chicken skewers are cooked, generously brush the reduced teriyaki sauce over the chicken pieces before serving.

128. Steamed Vegetarian Gyoza

 40 minutes

Nutritional Values (per single serving): Calories: about 150 kcal, Protein: about 4g, Carbohydrates: about 30g, Fat: about 1g, Fiber: about 2g, Sodium: 180mg

Ingredients:
- 6 gyoza wrappers
- 1 cup chopped napa cabbage
- 4 shiitake mushrooms, chopped
- 1 green onion, chopped
- 1 teaspoon freshly grated ginger
- 1 clove garlic, finely chopped
- 1 tablespoon low-sodium soy sauce

Instructions:
1. In a bowl, mix the chopped napa cabbage, chopped shiitake mushrooms, chopped green onion, grated ginger, and finely chopped garlic.
2. Take a gyoza wrapper and place a teaspoon of the vegetable mixture in the center.
3. Lightly moisten the edges of the wrapper with water and fold the wrapper in half over the filling, pressing the edges to seal well.
4. Repeat the process with the remaining wrappers and vegetable mixture until all ingredients are used.
5. Arrange the gyoza in a steaming basket, making sure to leave space between them to prevent sticking during cooking.
6. Steam the gyoza for about 10-12 minutes or until the wrapper becomes translucent and the filling is tender.
7. Serve the hot gyoza with low-sodium soy sauce for dipping.

129. Miso Soup with Tofu and Seaweed

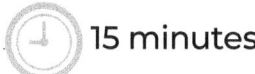 15 minutes

Nutritional Values (per single serving): Calories: about 150 kcal, Protein: about 10g, Carbohydrates: about 10g, Fat: about 8g, Fiber: about 3g, Sodium: 300mg

Ingredients:
- 1 cup dashi broth
- 50g tofu, diced
- 5g dried wakame seaweed
- 1 tablespoon miso
- 1 cup water

Instructions:
1. Bring the dashi broth to a boil in a pot.
2. Add the diced tofu and dried wakame seaweed to the boiling broth.
3. In a separate cup, dissolve the miso in a little water until smooth.
4. Add the diluted miso to the pot with the broth and mix well until completely dissolved.
5. Let the soup simmer for another 2-3 minutes to allow the flavors to meld.
6. Pour the hot miso soup into a bowl and serve immediately.

130. Japanese Ramen

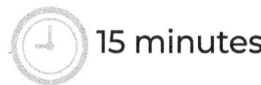 15 minutes

Nutritional Values (per single serving): Calories: about 150 kcal, Protein: about 10g, Carbohydrates: about 10g, Fat: about 8g, Fiber: about 3g, Sodium: 300mg

131. Miso Soup with Tofu and Seaweed (for one person)

Ingredients:
- 1 cup dashi broth
- 50g tofu, diced
- 5g dried wakame seaweed
- 1 tablespoon miso
- 1 cup water

Instructions:
1. Bring the dashi broth to a boil in a pot.
2. Add the diced tofu and dried wakame seaweed to the boiling broth.
3. In a separate cup, dissolve the miso in a little water until smooth.
4. Add the diluted miso to the pot with the broth and mix well until completely dissolved.
5. Let the soup simmer for another 2-3 minutes to allow the flavors to meld.
6. Pour the hot miso soup into a bowl and serve immediately.

Snack

132. Fruit Salad

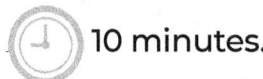 10 minutes.

Nutritional Values (per serving): Calories: about 80 kcal, Fiber: 4g, Sodium: 0mg, Badges: Vegan, Vegetarian.

Ingredients:
- Strawberries, blueberries, kiwi, pineapple, mango.

Instructions
1. Cut the fresh fruit into small pieces and mix gently. Serve the fruit salad in bowls or glasses.

133. Greek Yogurt with Blueberries and Almonds

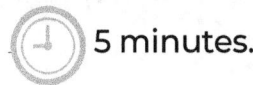 5 minutes.

Nutritional Values (per serving): Calories: about 150 kcal, Fiber: 2g, Sodium: 50mg, Badges: Vegetarian.

Ingredients:
- Low-fat Greek yogurt, fresh blueberries, almonds.

Instructions:
1. Pour the Greek yogurt into a bowl and add the fresh blueberries and sliced almonds as toppings.

134. Homemade Cereal Bars

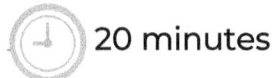 20 minutes

Nutritional Values (per bar): Calories: about 150 kcal, Protein: about 3g, Carbohydrates: about 15g, Fat: about 9g, Fiber: about 3g, Sodium: 50mg

Ingredients:
- 1 cup rolled oats
- 1/4 cup honey
- 1/4 cup peanut butter
- Chopped nuts of your choice (e.g., walnuts, almonds, hazelnuts)

Instructions:
1. In a saucepan over low heat, melt the honey and peanut butter until smooth.
2. Add the rolled oats and chopped nuts to the honey and peanut butter mixture. Stir well until all ingredients are incorporated.
3. Pour the mixture into a rectangular baking dish lined with parchment paper. Press down firmly with the back of a spoon or your hands to compact everything.
4. Let cool in the refrigerator for at least an hour, or until the bars have hardened.
5. Once the bars are well cooled and compact, cut them into individual bars.
6. Store the bars in an airtight container in the refrigerator to keep them fresh and crunchy.

135. Whole Grain Crackers with Avocado

 5 minutes

Nutritional Values (per serving of 2 crackers with avocado): Calories: about 120 kcal, Protein: about 2g, Carbohydrates: about 10g, Fat: about 8g, Fiber: about 3g, Sodium: 80mg

Ingredients:
- 2 whole grain crackers
- 1 ripe avocado
- Black pepper (to taste)

Instructions:
1. Cut the ripe avocado in half and remove the pit.
2. Mash the avocado flesh with a fork in a bowl until creamy.
3. Spread the mashed avocado evenly on the whole grain crackers.
4. Sprinkle black pepper over the spread avocado for an extra flavor kick.
5. Serve the whole grain crackers with avocado as a quick and healthy snack, rich in healthy fats and fiber.

136. Apple and Cinnamon Muffins

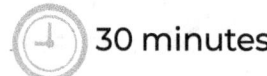 30 minutes

Nutritional Values (per muffin): Calories: about 150 kcal, Protein: about 3g, Carbohydrates: about 20g, Fat: about 6g, Fiber: about 3g, Sodium: 100mg

Ingredients:
- 1 cup whole wheat flour
- 1 grated apple
- 2 eggs
- 1/4 cup melted coconut oil
- 1 teaspoon ground cinnamon
- 1 teaspoon baking powder
- 1/4 cup brown sugar

Instructions:
1. Preheat the oven to 180°C (350°F) and prepare muffin tin with paper liners.
2. In a large bowl, mix together the whole wheat flour, cinnamon, and baking powder.
3. In another bowl, beat the eggs with the brown sugar and melted coconut oil until smooth.
4. Add the grated apple to the liquid mixture and mix well.
5. Gradually pour the dry ingredients into the bowl with the liquid mixture and mix until you get a smooth batter.
6. Distribute the batter into the muffin tins, filling them up to 3/4 of the capacity.
7. Bake the muffins in the preheated oven for about 20 minutes, or until they are golden brown and a toothpick inserted into the center comes out clean.
8. Once baked, let the muffins cool in the tin for a few minutes before transferring them to a wire rack to cool completely.
9. Serve the delicious apple and cinnamon muffins as a healthy snack or breakfast!

137. Chocolate Avocado Mousse

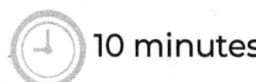 10 minutes

Nutritional Values (per serving): Calories: about 150 kcal, Protein: about 2g, Carbohydrates: about 12g, Fat: about 10g, Fiber: about 5g, Sodium: 20mg

Ingredients:
- 1 ripe avocado
- 2 tablespoons cocoa powder
- 1/4 cup almond milk
- 2 tablespoons maple syrup

Instructions:
1. In a blender or food processor, add the peeled and pitted ripe avocado.
2. Add the cocoa powder, almond milk, and maple syrup to the avocado.
3. Blend all the ingredients together until you get a creamy and smooth consistency.
4. Taste and add more maple syrup if you desire additional sweetness, adjusting to your personal preference.
5. Transfer the chocolate avocado mousse into small bowls or dessert glasses.
6. Place the bowls in the refrigerator for at least 30 minutes to slightly firm up the mousse and chill it.
7. Once the mousse has reached the desired consistency, serve cold and garnish with fresh fruit, chocolate shavings, or a dusting of cocoa powder, if desired.
8. Enjoy this delicious and creamy chocolate avocado mousse as a dessert or healthy indulgent snack!

138. Fruit and Nut Bars

 about 15-20 minutes plus chilling time in the refrigerator.

Nutritional Values (per bar): Calories: about 110 kcal, Protein: about 2g, Carbohydrates: about 12g, Fat: about 6g, Fiber: about 2g, Sodium: 0mg

Ingredients:
- 1 cup pitted dates
- 1 cup mixed nuts (walnuts, almonds, hazelnuts, etc.)
- 1/4 cup sunflower seeds
- 1/4 cup shredded coconut (optional)
- 1 teaspoon ground cinnamon (optional)

Instructions:
1. In a food processor, finely chop the pitted dates and mixed nuts until you get a sticky mixture.
2. Add the sunflower seeds to the mixture and mix well.
3. If desired, you can also add shredded coconut and cinnamon for an additional flavor boost.
4. Spread the mixture onto a parchment-lined baking sheet and press it down evenly with your hands.
5. Place the baking sheet in the refrigerator for at least an hour to firm up the mixture.
6. Once the mixture is solid, cut it into bars of desired size.
7. Store the bars in an airtight container in the refrigerator.

139. Peanut Butter and Rice Crispy Bars

 about 15-20 minutes plus chilling time in the refrigerator.

Nutritional Values (per bar): Calories: about 130 kcal, Protein: about 3g, Carbohydrates: about 12g, Fat: about 8g, Fiber: about 1g, Sodium: 50mg

Ingredients:
- 1 cup brown rice crispy cereal
- 1/2 cup natural peanut butter
- 1/4 cup honey or maple syrup
- 1 teaspoon vanilla extract
- A pinch of salt

Instructions:
1. In a large bowl, mix together the peanut butter, honey or maple syrup, vanilla extract, and salt until you get a homogeneous mixture.
2. Add the brown rice crispy cereal to the peanut butter mixture and gently mix until all the ingredients are well combined.
3. Transfer the mixture into a baking pan lined with parchment paper and press it down evenly with your hands or the back of a spoon.
4. Place the pan in the refrigerator for at least an hour or until the bars have firmed up.
5. Once the mixture is solidified, cut it into bars of the desired size.
6. Store the bars in an airtight container in the refrigerator.

Dessert

140. Banana and Cocoa Ice Cream

 10 minutes (plus additional freezing time).

Nutritional Values (per serving): Calories: about 120 kcal ,Protein: about 1g ,Carbohydrates: about 30g ,Fat: about 1g ,Fiber: about 4g ,Sodium: 1mg

Ingredients:
- Ripe bananas
- Unsweetened cocoa powder

Instructions:
1. Slice the ripe bananas into rounds and freeze them for at least 2 hours.
2. After the freezing period, place the banana slices in a blender along with the cocoa powder.
3. Blend the ingredients until you achieve a creamy and homogeneous consistency. If needed, you can add a little plant-based milk to aid in the blending process.
4. Transfer the banana and cocoa ice cream into a bowl and serve immediately.

141. Baked Pears with Cinnamon and Walnuts

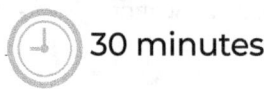 30 minutes

Nutritional Values (per serving): Calories: about 100 kcal ,Protein: about 1g ,Carbohydrates: about 20g ,Fat: about 3g ,Fiber: about 4g ,Sodium: 0mg

Ingredients:
- Ripe pears
- Ground cinnamon
- Chopped walnuts

Instructions:
1. Preheat the oven to 180°C and line a baking tray with parchment paper.
2. Cut the pears in half lengthwise and remove the seeds with a spoon.
3. Arrange the pear halves on the prepared baking tray with the cut side facing up.
4. Generously sprinkle the pears with ground cinnamon.
5. Evenly distribute the chopped walnuts over the pears.
6. Transfer the tray to the preheated oven and bake the pears for about 20-25 minutes, or until they become soft and slightly caramelized.
7. Once baked, remove the pears from the oven and let them cool slightly before serving.
8. Serve the baked pears warm, perhaps accompanied by a scoop of vanilla ice cream or with a drizzle of maple syrup if you desire an extra touch of sweetness.

142. Coconut and Mixed Berry Chia Pudding

 5 minutes (plus additional resting time).

Nutritional Values (per serving): Calories: about 150 kcal, Protein: about 3g, Carbohydrates: about 10g, Fat: about 11g, Fiber: about 8g, Sodium: 10mg

Ingredients:
- 1 cup coconut milk
- 2 tablespoons chia seeds
- Mixed berries (for garnish)

Instructions:
1. In a bowl, mix together the coconut milk and chia seeds until well combined.
2. Cover the bowl and let it rest in the refrigerator for at least 4 hours or preferably overnight. This will allow the chia seeds to absorb the liquid and form a pudding-like consistency.
3. Once the chia pudding has reached the desired consistency, remove it from the refrigerator and mix well.
4. Divide the chia pudding into servings and garnish with fresh mixed berries.
5. Serve chilled and enjoy this delicious coconut and mixed berry chia pudding as breakfast, snack, or dessert!

143. Sugar-Free Apple Cake

 45 minutes

Nutritional Values (per serving): Calories: about 120 kcal, Protein: about 2g, Carbohydrates: about 30g, Fat: about 1g, Fiber: about 4g, Sodium: 5mg

Ingredients:
- 3 apples
- 1 cup whole wheat flour
- 1 teaspoon ground cinnamon
- Juice of 1 lemon

Instructions:
1. Preheat the oven to 180°C (350°F) and prepare a lightly oiled or parchment paper-lined baking pan.
2. Peel the apples and slice them thinly. Arrange the apple slices in the prepared pan, overlapping them slightly if necessary.
3. Sprinkle the lemon juice over the apples and dust with cinnamon.
4. In a bowl, mix the whole wheat flour with a pinch of ground cinnamon.
5. Evenly sprinkle the flour mixture over the apples in the pan.
6. Bake the apple cake in the preheated oven for about 30-35 minutes or until the apples are tender and the top is lightly golden.
7. Once baked, let it cool slightly before serving.

144. Lemon Sorbet

 10 minutes (plus additional freezing time)

Nutritional Values (per serving): Calories: about 80 kcal ,Protein: about 1g ,Carbohydrates: about 22g ,Fat: about 0g ,Fiber: about 2g ,Sodium: 5mg

Ingredients:
- Juice of 4 lemons
- 1 cup water
- 1/4 cup agave syrup (or other sweetener of choice)

Instructions:
1. In a bowl, mix together freshly squeezed lemon juice, water, and agave syrup until well combined.
2. Pour the mixture into an ice cube tray or a shallow freezer-safe container.
3. Cover the tray or container with plastic wrap or a lid and place it in the freezer.
4. Let the sorbet freeze for about 4-6 hours, gently stirring every hour with a fork to break up ice crystals and achieve a creamier consistency.
5. Once the sorbet reaches the desired consistency, serve it in dessert bowls and garnish with lemon slices or fresh mint leaves, if desired.
6. Enjoy the refreshing and tangy lemon sorbet as a light and delicious dessert, perfect for summer days or as a refreshing end to a meal.

145. Coconut and Berry Panna Cotta

 15 minutes (plus additional cooling time)

Nutritional Values (per serving): Calories: about 120 kcal ,Protein: about 1g ,Carbohydrates: about 15g ,Fat: about 7g ,Fiber: about 3g ,Sodium: 10mg

Ingredients:
- 1 cup coconut milk
- 2 teaspoons agar agar powder
- 2 tablespoons maple syrup (or other sweetener of choice)
- Mixed berries for garnish

Instructions:
1. In a saucepan, bring coconut milk, maple syrup, and agar agar to a boil, stirring continuously to ensure the agar agar completely dissolves.
2. Once the mixture reaches boiling point, reduce the heat and let it simmer for another 2-3 minutes, stirring constantly, until it slightly thickens.
3. Pour the mixture into your preferred ramekins or molds.
4. Let it cool slightly at room temperature for about 10-15 minutes, then cover the molds with plastic wrap and transfer them to the refrigerator for at least 2 hours or until the panna cotta has completely set.
5. Once the coconut panna cotta is well chilled and set, gently unmold it onto dessert plates and garnish with a generous amount of mixed fresh berries.
6. Serve the coconut and berry panna cotta as an elegant and refreshing dessert, perfect for concluding a summer dinner or any special occasion. Enjoy!

146. Protein Banana Ice Cream

about 5 minutes plus freezing time

Nutritional Values (per serving): Calories: about 150 ,Protein: about 10g ,Carbohydrates: about 25g ,Fat: about 3g ,Fiber: about 4g ,Sodium: minimal

Ingredients:
- 2 ripe bananas, sliced and frozen
- 1/4 cup almond or coconut milk
- 1/2 teaspoon vanilla extract
- 1 tablespoon protein powder (of your choice)

Instructions:
1. In a blender or food processor, add the frozen bananas, almond or coconut milk, vanilla extract, and protein powder.
2. Blend the ingredients until smooth and creamy.
3. Transfer the protein ice cream mixture into a container and place it in the freezer for about 30 minutes to slightly firm up.
4. After freezing time, the protein ice cream will be ready to serve.
5. You can garnish the ice cream with a sprinkle of cinnamon or add some dark chocolate shavings for an extra flavor boost.
6. Serve the protein banana ice cream as a refreshing and nutritious dessert, perfect for enjoying after a workout or as a sweet treat any time of the day.

147. Fruit Crumble

about 15 minutes plus baking time

Nutritional Values (per serving): Calories: about 200 ,Protein: about 3g ,Carbohydrates: about 30g ,Fat: about 8g ,Fiber: about 6g ,Sodium: minimal

Ingredients:
- 2 cups mixed fruit (apples, pears, berries)
- Juice of half a lemon
- 1/2 cup rolled oats
- 2 tablespoons oat flour
- 2 tablespoons almond or coconut butter
- 1 tablespoon maple syrup or sweetener of choice

Instructions:
1. Preheat the oven to 180°C (350°F) and line a baking dish with parchment paper.
2. Chop the fruit into pieces and place them in a bowl. Add the lemon juice and mix well.
3. In another bowl, combine the rolled oats, oat flour, almond (or coconut) butter, and maple syrup until crumbly.
4. Pour the fruit into the prepared baking dish and sprinkle the crumble mixture on top.
5. Bake for about 25-30 minutes or until the crumble is golden and the fruit is soft.
6. Once baked, serve the warm crumble with a scoop of vanilla ice cream if you desire an extra touch of sweetness.
7. Enjoy this delicious dessert, perfect for a cozy evening or to finish a meal on a sweet and wholesome note.

148. Fruit Popsicles

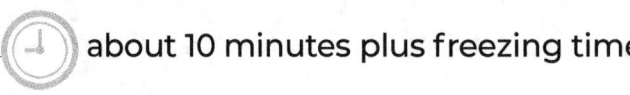 about 10 minutes plus freezing time

Nutritional Values (per popsicle): Calories: about 50 ,Protein: about 0.5g ,Carbohydrates: about 12g ,Fat: about 0.2g ,Fiber: about 2g ,Sodium: about 5mg

Ingredients:
- 2 cups mixed fruit (strawberries, blueberries, mango, etc.)
- 1/2 cup orange or apple juice
- 1 tablespoon maple syrup or sweetener of choice

Instructions:
1. Blend the fruit with the orange or apple juice and maple syrup until smooth.
2. Pour the mixture into popsicle molds.
3. Insert a stick into each mold and freeze for at least 4 hours or until solid.
4. Once frozen, quickly dip the molds in warm water to facilitate the removal of the popsicles.
5. Serve the fruit popsicles as a refreshing dessert. They are a delicious summer option, rich in fiber and low in calories, perfect for enjoying a guilt-free sweet treat.

Starred Dishes

149. Beetroot carpaccio with rocket salad and walnuts

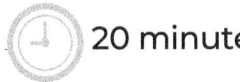 20 minutes

Nutritions: Calories: about 200 kcal, Protein: 3g, Fat: 15g, Carbohydrates: 15g, Fiber: 4g, Sodium: 90mg

Ingredients:
- Beetroot
- Rocket
- Walnuts
- Lemon juice
- Extra virgin olive oil

- Badges: Vegan, Vegetarian
- Difficulty: Easy. Requires minimal skills in beetroot preparation and ingredient arrangement.

Instructions:
• Beetroot Preparation: Thoroughly clean and peel the beetroot. Slice the beetroot thinly, preferably using a mandolin to get uniform slices.
• Carpaccio Assembly: Arrange the beetroot slices on a serving plate, slightly overlapping them. Squeeze some lemon juice over the beetroot slices and drizzle with extra virgin olive oil. Add a handful of fresh rocket over the beetroot.
• Rocket and Walnut Salad Preparation: In a bowl, mix rocket with roughly chopped walnuts. Dress the salad with some lemon juice and extra virgin olive oil.
• Plate Composition: Arrange the rocket and walnut salad over the beetroot slices. Complete the plate with some additional whole walnuts over the salad.
• Serving: Serve the Beetroot Carpaccio with Rocket Salad and Walnuts as an appetizer or as a light side dish.

150. Saffron Risotto with Asparagus and Parmesan Shavings

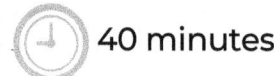 40 minutes

Nutritional Values (per serving): Calories: about 320 kcal, Protein: 9g, Fat: 7g, Carbohydrates: 55g, Fiber: 3g, Sodium: 300mg, Badge: Vegetarian

Ingredients:
- Arborio rice
- Saffron
- Asparagus
- Vegetable broth
- Onion
- White wine
- Parmesan cheese
- Difficulty: Medium. Requires skills in preparing risotto and cooking asparagus.

Instructions:
1. Asparagus Preparation: Clean the asparagus by removing the woody ends.
2. Cut the asparagus into pieces about 2-3 cm in length.
3. Broth Preparation: Heat the vegetable broth in a saucepan and keep it warm over low heat.
4. Saffron Preparation: In a small bowl, place the saffron and add a couple of tablespoons of hot broth. Let it infuse.
5. Risotto Preparation: In a large pot, sauté finely chopped onion in a little olive oil until translucent.
6. Add Arborio rice and toast for a couple of minutes, stirring constantly.
7. Deglaze with white wine and let the alcohol evaporate.
8. Gradually add the warm vegetable broth, one ladle at a time, stirring occasionally and waiting for it to be absorbed before adding more.
9. After about 15 minutes, add the asparagus to the rice and continue cooking until the risotto is creamy and the asparagus is tender but still crispy.
10. Adding Saffron: Add the infused saffron to the risotto and mix well until the color and flavor are uniform.
11. Finishing and Serving: Turn off the heat and keep the saffron and asparagus risotto warm.
12. Add a generous sprinkle of grated Parmesan cheese and gently mix.
13. Distribute the risotto onto serving plates and garnish with some fresh Parmesan shavings.
14. Serve immediately and enjoy this delicious risotto dish!
15. This recipe offers a creamy and fragrant risotto, enriched with the flavor of asparagus and the luxurious touch of saffron and Parmesan cheese.

151. Grilled Salmon with Ginger Lime Sauce

Full Nutritional Values (per serving):

Nutritions: Calories: about 250 kcal, Protein: about 25g, Fat: about 15g, Carbohydrates: about 3g, Fiber: about 1g, Sodium: about 100mg

Ingredients (for one person):
- 1 salmon fillet
- 1 tablespoon freshly grated ginger
- Juice of 1 lime
- 1 clove garlic
- finely chopped
- 1 fresh chili pepper
- thinly sliced
- Salt and pepper to taste

Instructions:
1. Preparing the Ginger Lime Sauce: Grate the fresh ginger until you have about 1 tablespoon of grated ginger.
2. In a bowl, mix the lime juice with the finely chopped garlic and sliced fresh chili pepper.
3. Add the grated ginger to the mixture and season with salt and pepper. Mix well and taste to adjust the flavor, if needed.
4. Marinating the Salmon: Place the salmon fillet in a shallow dish or a food storage bag.
5. Pour the ginger lime sauce over the salmon fillet, making sure to coat it well on all sides.
6. Cover the dish or seal the bag and let it marinate in the refrigerator for at least 20 minutes.
7. Grilling the Salmon: Preheat the grill to medium-high heat and lightly brush with olive oil to prevent the fish from sticking.
8. Once the grill is hot, place the salmon fillet on the grill and cook for about 4-5 minutes per side, flipping it once with a spatula for even cooking.
9. Ensure the salmon is thoroughly cooked but still tender and juicy on the inside.
10. Finishing and Serving: Once cooked, transfer the grilled salmon to a serving plate.
11. Drizzle some fresh lime juice over the salmon before serving.
12. You can accompany the salmon with fresh sides, such as a mixed salad or basmati rice.
13. This recipe offers a fresh and flavorful salmon dish, enhanced by the vibrant ginger lime sauce.

152. Saffron Risotto with Asparagus and Parmesan Shavings

Full Nutritional Values (per serving): Calories: about 320 kcal, Protein: about 8g, Fat: about 7g, Carbohydrates: about 57g, Fiber: about 3g, Sodium: about 300mg

Ingredients (for one person):

- 70g Arborio rice
- 100g asparagus
- 1/4 onion
- 1/2 glass dry white wine
- 300ml vegetable broth
- 1 sachet saffron
- Extra virgin olive oil
- Salt and pepper to taste
- Parmesan shavings for serving

Instructions:

1. Preparing the Ingredients: Finely chop the onion.
2. Cut the asparagus into pieces, removing the tough ends.
3. Sautéing the Onion and Toasting the Rice: In a pot, heat a drizzle of olive oil over medium heat.
4. Add the onion and let it soften slightly.
5. Add the Arborio rice and lightly toast it for about 2-3 minutes, stirring continuously.
6. Deglazing with White Wine: Pour the dry white wine into the toasted rice and onion.
7. Stir and let the alcohol evaporate, continuing to stir until the wine is completely absorbed.
8. Preparing the Saffron and Adding to the Broth: In a small container, add the saffron to a small amount of hot broth and stir until the saffron has dissolved completely.
9. Add the rest of the vegetable broth to the pot with the rice and onion.
10. Adding Asparagus and Cooking the Risotto: Add the chopped asparagus to the rice in the pot.
11. Mix well and let the risotto cook over medium-low heat, gradually adding broth as needed, stirring occasionally, until the rice is al dente and has reached a creamy consistency. This should take about 18-20 minutes.
12. Serving: Ensure the asparagus is tender and the rice is creamy but still al dente.
13. Adjust with salt and pepper to taste.
14. Serve the risotto hot, garnishing each portion with generous shavings of fresh Parmesan cheese.

153. Vegetable Flan with Light Cheese Fondue

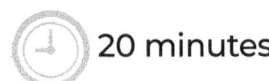 20 minutes 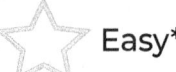 Easy*

*Requires minimal skills in preparing and cutting the vegetables and arranging the ingredients.

Full Nutritional Values (per serving): Calories: about 200 kcal, Protein: about 4g, Fat: about 15g, Carbohydrates: about 15g, Fiber: about 4g, Sodium: about 90mg

Ingredients:
- 2 medium beetroots
- 2 handfuls of arugula
- 1/4 cup of walnuts, toasted and chopped
- Juice of 1 lemon
- 2 tablespoons of extra virgin olive oil
- Salt and freshly ground black pepper

Instructions:
1. Preparing the Beetroots: Remove the ends of the beetroots and peel them.
2. Slice the beetroots into very thin slices, preferably using a mandoline slicer to achieve uniform slices.
3. Preparing the Dressing: In a small bowl, mix the lemon juice with the extra virgin olive oil.
4. Season with salt and freshly ground black pepper according to your taste.
5. Assembling the Carpaccio: Arrange the beetroot slices in a single layer on a serving plate.
6. Dress the beetroot slices with the prepared lemon and olive oil dressing.
7. Preparing the Arugula and Walnut Salad: Place the arugula on top of the dressed beetroot slices.
8. Sprinkle the chopped walnuts over the salad.
9. Serving: Serve the beetroot carpaccio with arugula and walnut salad immediately to maintain the freshness and crispness of the ingredients.

154. Tuna Tartare with Guacamole

Full Nutritional Values (per serving): Calories: about 280 kcal, Protein: about 18g, Fat: about 20g, Carbohydrates: about 14g, Fiber: about 9g, Sodium: about 350mg

Ingredients (for one person):

- 150g fresh tuna
- Juice of 1 lime
- 1 tablespoon low-sodium soy sauce
- 1/2 tablespoon sesame oil
- 1/2 chopped chili pepper
- 1 ripe avocado
- 1 diced tomato
- 1/8 chopped red onion
- 1 tablespoon chopped fresh cilantro
- Juice of 1/2 lime
- Salt to taste
- Crispy corn chips, for serving

Instructions:

1. Preparing the Tuna Tartare: Dice the fresh tuna and place it in a bowl.
2. Season the tuna with lime juice, low-sodium soy sauce, sesame oil, and chopped chili pepper. Mix well and let it marinate for at least 10 minutes.
3. Preparing the Guacamole: Mash the ripe avocado in a bowl.
4. Add diced tomato, chopped red onion, chopped fresh cilantro, chopped chili pepper, and lime juice to the bowl. Mix everything well.
5. Adjust the salt according to your taste.
6. Serving: Arrange the marinated tuna tartare on a serving plate.
7. Serve with a generous portion of guacamole.
8. Serve with crispy corn chips.

155. Soy Glazed Salmon with Ginger Lime Sauce and Crispy Salad

 30 minutes

Nutritional Values: Protein: 25g, Fiber: 5g, Calories: 320, Sodium: 350mg, Badges: Fish, Gluten-Free, Low Sodium

Ingredients:

- 2 fresh salmon fillets
- 3 tablespoons low-sodium soy sauce
- 1 tablespoon honey or maple syrup
- Juice of 1 lime
- 1 teaspoon freshly grated ginger
- 2 cloves garlic, minced
- 2 tablespoons olive oil
- Salt and freshly ground black pepper
- 4 cups crispy lettuce (such as romaine lettuce), washed and chopped
- 1 cucumber, thinly sliced
- 1 grated carrot
- 1/4 cup sliced almonds, toasted
- Sesame seeds for garnish

INSTRUCTIONS:

1. Preheat the oven to 200°C and line a baking sheet with parchment paper.
2. In a small bowl, mix together the soy sauce, honey, lime juice, grated ginger, and minced garlic.
3. Place the salmon fillets on the prepared baking sheet and generously brush with the soy sauce mixture.
4. Bake the salmon in the preheated oven for about 12-15 minutes, or until the salmon is cooked through and flakes easily with a fork.
5. Meanwhile, prepare the crispy salad: In a large bowl, combine the lettuce, sliced cucumber, grated carrot, and toasted almonds.
6. Dress the salad with olive oil, salt, and pepper.
7. Once cooked, remove the salmon from the oven and serve hot accompanied by the crispy salad.
8. Finish the dish by sprinkling the salmon with sesame seeds and adding a lime wedge for a final touch of freshness.

156. Chicken Breast Stuffed with Spinach and Ricotta with Mashed Potatoes and Sautéed Asparagus

Nutritional Values (per serving): Protein: about 35g ,Carbohydrates: about 30g ,Fat: about 18g ,Fiber: about 6g Calories: about 380 ,Sodium: about 320mg

Ingredients (for one person):

- 1 boneless, skinless chicken breast
- 1/2 cup fresh spinach, washed and chopped
- 1/4 cup ricotta cheese
- 1 tablespoon grated Parmesan cheese
- 1 clove garlic, minced
- 1/2 tablespoon olive oil
- Salt and freshly ground black pepper, to taste
- 250g potatoes, peeled and cubed
- 125g asparagus, washed and trimmed
- 1 tablespoon butter
- Chopped fresh parsley for garnish

Instructions:

1. **Preheat the Oven:** Preheat the oven to 180°C.
2. **Prepare the Spinach and Ricotta Filling:** In a bowl, mix the chopped spinach, ricotta cheese, grated Parmesan cheese, minced garlic, salt, and pepper.
3. **Prepare the Chicken Breast:** Make a horizontal incision on the chicken breast to create a pocket, being careful not to cut all the way through. Fill the chicken breast pocket with the spinach and ricotta mixture.
4. Cook the Chicken Breast:
   - Heat olive oil in a non-stick skillet over medium-high heat.
   - Add the chicken breast and cook for 6-7 minutes per side, or until golden brown and cooked through.
5. Prepare the Mashed Potatoes:
   - Meanwhile, cook the potatoes in boiling salted water until tender.
   - Drain well and mash with butter, salt, and pepper.
6. Prepare the Sautéed Asparagus:
   - Cut the asparagus into 5 cm pieces and sauté them in a skillet with a little olive oil, salt, and pepper until tender but still crisp.
7. Assemble the Plate:
   - Arrange the stuffed chicken breast on a serving plate.
   - Serve with mashed potatoes and sautéed asparagus.
8. Garnish and Serve:
   - Garnish with chopped fresh parsley before serving.

CONCLUSION

In conclusion, this cookbook offers a wide range of recipes specifically designed to meet the tastes and needs of individuals affected by fatty liver disease. We understand the importance of adopting a balanced and targeted diet to manage this condition, and we hope that the recipes presented can provide inspiration and support in creating delicious and healthy meals.

Each recipe has been carefully developed taking into account recommended and discouraged foods for fatty liver disease, ensuring a balance between taste, nutritional value, and practicality. We have included options for breakfast, lunch, dinner, snacks, and desserts, thus offering a variety of dishes for every occasion.

Furthermore, we have included detailed information on the nutritional values of each recipe, including levels of sodium and fiber, to allow for conscious and informed choices. "Vegan" and "vegetarian" badges have been added to facilitate the search for recipes suitable for different dietary styles.

If you have enjoyed our culinary creations, we would be grateful if you could leave a review to share your opinion with other food enthusiasts like yourself. Thank you for your support!

We hope that this cookbook can be a useful tool for those seeking to adopt a healthy and balanced diet while managing fatty liver disease. Always remember to consult your doctor or a dietitian before making significant changes to your diet. Bon appétit and good health!